THE PETiTE ADVANTAGE DIET

Also by Jim Karas

The 7-Day Energy Surge

The Cardio-Free Diet

Flip the Switch

The Business Plan for the Body

THE
PETiTE
ADVANTAGE
DIET

Achieve That Long, Lean Look.
The Specialized Plan for Women
5'4" and Under.

Jim Karas

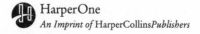
HarperOne
An Imprint of HarperCollins*Publishers*

HarperOne

THE PETITE ADVANTAGE DIET: *Achieve That Long, Lean Look. The Specialized Plan for Women 5'4" and Under.* Copyright © 2011 by Jim Karas. All rights reserved. Printed in the United States of America. No part of this book may be used or reproduced in any manner whatsoever without written permission except in the case of brief quotations embodied in critical articles and reviews. For information, address HarperCollins Publishers, 10 East 53rd Street, New York, NY 10022.

HarperCollins books may be purchased for educational, business, or sales promotional use. For information, please e-mail the Special Markets Department at SPsales@harpercollins.com.

HarperCollins website: http://www.harpercollins.com

HarperCollins®, ▄▄®, and HarperOne™ are trademarks of HarperCollins Publishers.

FIRST HARPERCOLLINS PAPERBACK EDITION PUBLISHED IN 2013

Designed by Terry McGrath

Library of Congress Cataloging-in-Publication Data is available upon request.

ISBN 978-0-06-202546-3

13 14 15 16 17   RRD(H)   10 9 8 7 6 5 4 3 2 1

*To my two
personal Petites,
my children,
Olivia and Evan.*

CONTENTS

INTRODUCTION

Back in 1986, one of my first personal training clients was a 5'4" 32-year-old woman who weighed 145 pounds. Like so many women I have encountered, she just wanted to lose twenty pounds to get back to 125, which she felt was her ideal weight.

Another 5'3" 41-year-old woman, hovering around 170 pounds, had weighed in the mid-130s for around the past twenty years. But after two daughters, a divorce, and a demanding job, she felt it was virtually impossible to shed even one pound.

One of my favorite clients was a 5'1" 56-year-old woman who told me she would be happy weighing *anything* under 200 pounds. She went so far as to say she would be thrilled if the weight *gain* would just stop! She was a lifelong struggler with some serious health issues and so discouraged that she was ready to just throw in the towel. FYI, she was one of my favorite Petites because she fought hard to lose the weight—and she won!

When I look back over my twenty-five years as a weight-loss and fitness professional—now, after four books, they actually call me an expert!—I realize that I have heard the same complaints over and over from shorter women, whom I will lovingly refer to as Petites:

- I can't lose weight. My husband diets for a week and loses ten pounds. I drop a quarter-pound if I'm lucky.

- Susan eats all the foods I never get to eat and rarely gains weight. If she does gain weight, it's gone in a flash. I wonder if that's because she's 5'9"?

- Many of my taller friends don't exercise and I am at it all the time. They stay slim and I gain weight. What's wrong with me? (Flash bulletin—the most popular form of exercise, cardio, actually makes most people *gain* weight. Is that you?)

Here is how I answer these complaints:

1. There is nothing wrong with you.

2. When it comes to weight loss, Petites require a customized plan.

And that is what this book is all about.

Why do Petites require a different plan? Well, start with these statistics:

- 68 percent of American adults are overweight and 34 percent are obese. In 1960, these figures were 45 and 13 percent respectively. That's a *huge* increase (and don't even think about blaming your genes!).

- One-third of children and adolescents are overweight and 20 percent are obese (only 4 percent were obese in 1960). I will explain why this is important later in this introduction.

- Americans now consume 2700 calories a day, about 500 more than they did forty years ago.[1] Simply put, more calories will equal more weight, especially for those of a shorter stature.

> **While I realize the theme of this book is weight loss,** I hope that I can convince you to discover that, along with most weight loss, comes improved overall health, more energy, a slowing if not stalling of the aging process, and a host of other benefits to your mind and body. Research proves that just a 10 percent reduction in your body weight results in more sex—sounds good to me! I know it sounds trite, but I finish almost every speech I give with the line: "You only get one mind and one body. Why not give it the very, very best?" I hope you know that, believe that, and respect your one mind and one body—because you aren't getting another one.

Petites, stop for a moment and truly ask yourselves: "Can I really lose weight?" Here are the two answers I've heard in the past:

- Probably a few pounds, but nowhere near what I want to in order to really like my body (and it would probably be *really* hard).

- Honestly, no. I just can't lose weight.

And I bet you are reading this and thinking: "Right, so what do I do?" Stay tuned, I have a results-producing weight-loss plan for you, and only you. And, you'll see that your smaller stature actually becomes an *advantage*.

So, let's stop thinking about your height as something you need to overcome and start thinking about how to use it to your advantage. Let's first tackle your belief system.

In the past, you were probably following a plan that was meant for the general population, which includes a lot of people taller than you are. If you had been following my plan, you would have seen results. So, just for now, until I lay out the program for you, cling to the belief that you absolutely *will* lose weight this time. To help you do that, I am going to wrap your head around the results-producing mind-set that is essential to—you guessed it—getting results! They go hand in hand. Sure, the goal is to get you to "take action," but we can't accomplish that until I positively tinker with your mind. Only with a "new and improved" belief system can you adopt the new behaviors necessary to achieve a different outcome—a.k.a. weight loss. That is what chapter 1, "Selfish Is Good," is all about. I bet you always thought that putting others first was a virtue. No, no, no. You will soon learn that when you are selfish, everyone around you benefits *and* you lose weight.

The Numbers

Petites, I am going to "start your engines" for weight loss by helping you optimize your metabolism and the calories you burn—not just during exercise, but twenty-four hours a day, seven days a week. You can increase your metabolism at any age; it's never too late. That's why chapter 2 is entitled "Metabolism: Your Weapon of Mass Reduction." In chapter 2, we'll dissect the word "metabolism" and clear up a lot of confusion, setting the record straight that a pumping metabolism is your first essential component to successful, long-term weight loss.

Look back for a moment and focus on the last bullet point on page 2. Americans are consuming 500 more calories a day than they did forty years ago. If you happen to be a vertically enhanced (taller) person who requires approximately 2500 calories a day to maintain your weight, then 500 *more* calories a day represents a 20 percent increase. But if you are a Petite who requires only 1600 calories a day, then 500 more calories a day represents over a 31 percent increase in calories. (Don't be surprised by that number, ladies. If you are moderately sedentary—as in little or no activity or exercise—it is probably close to your reality.) Ouch! That's what chapter 3, "The Math," is all about. If you work the math, you will finally understand why you must operate under different assumptions (like the fact that you *can't* eat like the big girls) when it comes to weight loss.

Have you ever wondered why they make clothes for Petites but not food? Well, since it's probably not going to happen anytime soon, I'm going to teach you in chapter 4 how to think like a Petite when it comes to selecting the right food that tastes good—in appropriate portions with the least amount of calories. Plus, I'm going to show you how to get the biggest nutritional/metabolic-boosting bang from each bite. And I'm going to introduce you to the word "satiety."

Satiety is simply defined as a feeling of fullness. Think of it as a derivative of the word "satisfied." You can literally teach your body, through actions and hormones, how to feel full on fewer calories, because that is what your smaller body needs.

I know, I know; you don't want to hear that you have to count calories, but relax and breathe because I'm going to do it for you. (FYI, deep breathing is very helpful if your goal is weight loss, because it reduces stress hormones that tell your body to store fat.) By choosing the right combination of foods and eating them at the right time of day, you will enhance your satiety mechanisms and not feel hungry. Hunger is your enemy and, let's be honest, who wants to spend the rest of their life hungry—and cranky? I don't. By following this very specific eating plan, you won't. There are a number of ways to enhance satiety and doing so is the key to your successful permanent weight loss. Embrace the feeling of being satisfied, because you can use this to your advantage.

The Eating Plan

Once you believe you can lose weight and understand the math of weight loss, I'll explain certain components of your eating plan. We will explore certain calorie-blasting foods—like the right proteins and spices (surprised?)—and certain calorie-blasting behaviors—like eating breakfast. I know you have probably heard this before, but the more you understand *why* I am instructing you to eat and do certain things, the more you will be committed to living this plan. I want you to *understand* this plan and not just follow it. That puts you in the driver's seat and not the passenger seat. Drivers generally determine the way to get where they want to go! I'm going to turn you into a driver and teach you how to avoid potholes (lack of planning), excessive traffic (huge portions), and other out-of-control drivers (a saboteur, such as a so-called friend insanely jealous of the longer, leaner you) you may encounter on the road to permanent weight loss. Drivers lead the way! And you're going to be a leader.

Just as there are foods and behaviors I want you to embrace, there are also certain foods and behaviors I want you to avoid. Three words that I will introduce you to in chapter 4 are "in addition to." Petites must eliminate or seriously minimize "in addition to" foods, which I call "Addies." A simple example is salad dressing. I'll teach you how to whip up a great-tasting, satisfying dressing that doesn't contain a lot of calories. I have achieved great success for Petites by moving them away from traditional salad dressings. By just reducing the calories from Addies right away, you will quickly start to experience weight loss.

Addies, for Petites, can make the difference between carrying extra pounds and being lean. As a Petite, you simply don't have the body size to "stomach" these additional calories— literally. Learning to enjoy food and learning how to find it satisfying will free your taste buds and set you on the path to a leaner, sexier you. And this one change is so easy to do. Right now, you are probably in the habit of using Addies regularly and then saying to yourself: "Why can't I lose any weight?" The answer may be sitting right there on top of your lettuce and inside your sautéed spinach. I'm going to teach you what ingredients to use and exactly the right amount that your body needs—and that your brain likes.

Next comes the actual twenty-one-day Eating Plan, which provides you with exact portions, recipes, and shopping lists. Carbohydrates (carbs) will be explained in a startling new way and will not be vilified as they have been for the last decade. Carbs are a Petite's secret weapon. Knowing how to eat carbs correctly and knowing which carbs are best will keep you losing weight. Once you master carbs, you will lose more fat than ever before by cycling calories and carbs in and out of your daily caloric intake in a very specific pattern. Chapter 5 is filled with what you finally need to know to make weight loss happen while staying full, hormonally balanced, and happy.

Bet you never experienced that "trifecta" before when dieting!

Then, just when you are ready to sail into the "Land of the Lean," you get slammed with a headwind—eating out. Restaurants know that the majority of their patrons want a lot of value for their money. Sure, value is important, but it doesn't have to mean the "end of lean." Chapter 6 gives you tools to enjoy breakfast, lunch, or dinner out and *not* suffer deprivation or major caloric damage. You are even allowed to eat out during the critical first twenty-one days of my Advantage plan. I will tell you exactly what to order in each type of restaurant, whether it is Italian, Mexican, Chinese, Greek, or a steak house. Most of the Petites I work with are initially petrified to eat out, especially when they are shedding a lot of weight and fat on my plan while eating at home. Once I teach them what to do, they are relieved and happy that they don't have to come up with more lame excuses for dodging dinners out.

Here's a tease. Everyone is talking about the benefits of olive oil, but too much will pack on the pounds. Did you know that olive oil is 120 calories per tablespoon and 100 percent fat? So *please*, immediately stop pouring it all over your food and, if you use it (which I do allow in the eating plan), then use it smartly and sparingly. Many years ago, I coined the phrase: "Shine and glimmer won't make you slimmer." Petites, if the food is shining back at you, especially when you are eating out, put the fork down, because this food is probably packed with calories that you don't need and probably don't even want.

Did you know that the vast majority of Petites totally sabotage their weight-loss plan by what they drink? Yep, liquid calories are predominantly evil (the poison the wicked step-mother offered you was less lethal than juice—at least when it comes to weight loss!). Beverages are platinum members of the Addies club. There are exceptions, however—delicious drinks that I present in chapter 7 that will keep you hydrated and on point while you drop the pounds. Here's a hint: Did you know that a glass of wine and a cup of tea both give you a metabolic bump?

Exercise

I call chapter 8 "Exercise: A Petite's BFF." You absolutely, positively *must* exercise, but you only have to start with a touch more than an hour and a half—a week! That's just three thirty-one-minute sessions (I'll explain why thirty-one minutes is key), for a total of an hour and thirty-three minutes a week. Forget the unrealistic hour a day. Who has the time, energy, or desire to do that? I will teach you the absolute best way to use your smaller frame in a way that not only slims your body super fast, but also sheds inches from your midsection.

You will never, ever have to get on a treadmill, elliptical trainer, stair stepper, or bike again and you'll learn that cardio is the perfect way for Petites to *gain* weight. Yep, if you want to pile on the pounds (lots of research agrees that cardio does nothing but make you hungry), stress out your joints and body, gain weight in your midsection, ruin your posture, speed up the aging process, and feel totally depleted of energy, then lace up those running shoes and hit the pavement. Of course you don't want to do that, so chapter 8 will enlighten you.

Here's another major plus to my exercise program. For the first time in your life, you are going to experience what I call a body "reconfiguration." Your whole body will be transformed, as this program is not just about weight loss. It's about *fat* loss and sculpting the proportions of your body. See, being a Petite gives you the perfect landscape to accomplish this goal. Taller gals can't achieve the same perfect proportions that you can. I know you may envy those Amazon-like supermodels, but ask yourself if you would rather look like Reese Witherspoon, Kelly Ripa, Penelope Cruz, Jada Pinkett Smith, Salma Hayek, Natalie Portman, or Dolly Parton. These ladies span more than three decades and, once again, prove that you can be a very sexy, lean Petite. All you require is the right program—this one!

I want to be perfectly clear one more time about this critical point; we are 100 percent in the *fat-loss* business. We are going to maintain consistent water levels and hold onto muscle at all costs while we blast fat off your body. Again, this is your first body "recomposition." We are going to shed lots of fat while increasing your metabolism and create a whole new-and-improved body as well as a whole new enlightened mind-set to go with that body. Trust me; this exercise program will be different from anything you have done in the past. I know I have alluded to the true advantage of this plan before, but this exercise program will literally blow your mind while blowing off your fat.

Want to lose five pounds in the next five seconds?
Pull your shoulders and chin back, tuck in your abs, and sit up straight. While I feel posture is important to everyone, it is imperative for Petites. By standing tall, you look better, feel more confident, and immediately lean out your abs. A small midsection is how I can help you look smaller and better proportioned. Millions of books have been written about flattening your abs; how many weight-loss titles have the word "abs" right in the title? But they don't work. They don't work because they don't know how to lean out your abs and midsection. I do. It's a combination of things, not just one kind of crunch—which, FYI, is a useless exercise to reduce your midsection—or one kind of food. It's about putting a comprehensive plan into action.

I know you've probably tried other weight-loss plans in the past, dropped a _few_ pounds, but ultimately ended up hitting that dreaded word—plateau. I promise you that is not going to happen this time, as you will lose all the weight you desire. You never will hit those dreaded, frustrating plateaus, because I will teach you the concept of "progression." You see, your body will listen to what you tell it to do. It's very, very smart. But you have to keep challenging your body and thereby _forcing_ it to change. That will come from changing up your exercise program. You'll learn the complete program in chapter 8, then start to see the changes in chapter 9. Part of the progression comes from just an increase in intensity. And because you are a Petite, your smaller stature allows you to work out harder without risking injury. That's a major advantage for you that I bet you never knew. You have this great advantage because you are smaller, lower to the ground, and more compact. So, in chapter 8, I will show you simple changes to your exercise program that will make "plateau" a word from the past.

This book will give you:

- A new way to believe in weight loss

- A rockin' metabolism

- The math of weight loss

- The science behind my eating and exercise program, *plus* the actual program.

Your Environment

Next, you need to assess your environment. When was the last time you felt you truly had a partner in a mission? Some of you may be fortunate enough to have a terrific spouse, partner, BFF, family member, or co-worker, but is he or she the best partner for you when it comes to taking off the pounds? In chapter 9, I'll help you identify your BFF specifically for this plan. Why? Well, by having the right partner, you increase your chances of success from 24 to 66 percent.[2] That's a *huge* advantage! Plus, new research conclusively shows that the people you hang around with have an enormous impact on your body weight.

In addition to identifying a weight-loss partner, I implore you to examine the environment you place yourself in every day. Are you living in what the CDC (Centers for Disease Control and Prevention) refers to as an "obesogenic" environment that promotes increased food intake, unhealthy food choices, and physical inactivity? There is even startling new research from Tufts University showing how certain brains behave when they see, smell, or even hear the word "cake" or other similar, pleasurable foods. They light

> **Calling all moms!** Here's another motivator to get you to embrace weight loss. According to a 2009 study, females whose mothers were overweight have a ten-fold risk of being obese as adults. That's why I earlier sited the research about the frightening increase in weight gain and obesity in children. Ladies, that means that taking control of your weight will benefit both you and your daughters, especially if you partner up. And that benefit will probably trickle down to other young, impressionable girls around you.[4]

up the way alcoholics do when they see alcohol.[3] Knowing that your brain is literally going to "light up" when it even sees high-calorie or high-sugar goods, you need to make strategic plans about with whom and where you are going to eat. Should you choose to go to your favorite restaurant where you know you can't resist the double-chocolate upside-down cake? And should you go with a friend, family member, or co-worker who you know won't resist it either? I hope you realize the answer to this is "no," except on special, rare occasions.

So, let's assume you are eating and drinking right, exercising, standing up straighter, and have found the perfect partner with whom to shed the weight. What else can you do? I call chapter 10 "The Bag of Tricks," as there are actually a lot of things you can and should do (like sleep, breathe, and meditate, to name a few) to make this whole process easier, more effective, less stressful, and enjoyable. When was the last time the word "enjoyable" was used in a sentence regarding weight loss?

Be proud of being a Petite, as there are many advantages to "Petiteness":

- More mates to choose from. Hey Tom Cruise, Robert Redford, and Jon Stewart, it's me! And you look tall!

- Smaller, sexier feet. Excuse me, Mr. Blahnik and Mr. Choo, I'm ready for my close-up!

- Longer life. There is startling research demonstrating that Petites live longer, and some even possess a gene linked to longevity. Don't you just feel sorry for the stressed-out, pumping hearts of those long, "leggy" runway models? Why do you think they're sneering all the time?

- Reduced risk of cardiovascular disease and cancer. Did you know that more women die each year from cardiovascular disease than men? Being a Petite reduces that risk. Ditto for cancer.

- Less back and joint pain. Smaller people endure less back pain because of gravity (they don't have to reach as far down to take groceries out of the trunk) and possess shorter limbs, which reduces the risk of shoulder, neck, and elbow pain. Do I hear limbo party?

- Ability to work out much harder and more safely. Petites possess stronger muscles in proportion to body weight, which also translates into faster reaction times, greater endurance, and minimal joint pain.

By now, you may be thinking: "Why am I, a Petite, going to take weight-loss advice from a six-foot-tall man?" Well, here are four answers I have for you:

1. I understand you. As I said in the beginning of this introduction, my first experience as a weight-loss professional was with Petites. Had they *not* lost weight, my business would never

have grown so successfully and, clearly, I would not be writing this book. I have helped thousands of Petites lose weight.

2. My work is research-based. Almost everything I will tell you to do in this plan is supported by research. If something I say is what I call a "Karasism"— an observation or experience that is not supported by research, but rather by my own results—I will tell you.

3. I'm not going to rest until you are a success. The word "tenacious" has been used to describe me for as long as I can remember. I won't let you quit; I won't let you get discouraged; I won't let you stay at a weight at which you are not happy. As your guide, I will get you to your ultimate destination.

4. I've been there. I was an overweight child and young adult. I know how hard it is just to get started, and then actually to stick with a plan. But I also know how amazing it feels to take back control over your mind and body.

So, here it is, just for you. This is the first comprehensive weight-loss plan specifically written for Petites. The key to this plan's success is putting it all together, which I will help you do. Many of the tips in this book offer just a *slight* increase in metabolism (like drinking tea and spicing up your food), or just a *few* extra calories burned (by exercising in the most effective way and getting out of your chair), or an *optimized* hormonal balance for weight loss (through sleep and reduced stress). While many researchers have historically downplayed the effects of these simple techniques on weight loss, for Petites, every possible additional calorie burned is essential to success. It's a bit like compound interest; a little here and a little there and you end up "the millionaire next door." My goal is to make you the "skinny-mini bitch" next door.

CHAPTER 1 SELFISH IS GOOD!

Is that the first time you have ever heard that phrase? I believe wholeheartedly in being selfish when it comes to caring for yourself and I also believe that being selfish and placing yourself first is critically important to your success at weight loss.

For the past five years, I have been speaking at Oprah's live magazine events called "O You!" The events promote Oprah's "live your best life" message and include all of her contributors and favorites, like Suze Orman, Nate Berkus, Dr. Mehmet Oz (I've been on his show a number of times and he's a great guy), Martha Beck, and Stacy London, to name a few. When I first prepared my speech, I hadn't touched upon this concept of "selfish is good." It wasn't until I kept hammering another phrase—"put yourself first and everyone benefits; put yourself first and everyone benefits"—that one of the women raised her hand (she was actually a Petite) and said: "But isn't that selfish?" To which I replied: "Yes, but selfish is *good!* Selfish is *smart.* Selfish is what makes you live your best life, because you are giving yourself the best *first* and that will enable you to give your best back to others." The women cheered, loudly.

I don't know where it came from, but I just blurted it out and it resonated immediately with the audience and with me. The event became a bit like a rock concert and I actually made them stand up and chant with me: "Selfish is good; selfish is smart!"

This is the first belief system I want you to work on. The old belief is: "Everything and everyone else comes first and I come last." You believed, in the past, that:

- Your family comes first.

- Your home comes first.

- Your aging/ill parents, siblings, or friends come first.

- Your job comes first.

- Your church and community responsibilities come first.

Let's examine that for a moment. You are the cog that holds all these moving parts in place, yet you assign to yourself little or no value. Are you supposed to just pick up whatever crumb of time is left over to make a better food choice, to sleep, to exercise, to breathe, to do whatever is required to take care of yourself (and lose weight) so that you can then take care of everyone and everything else? Do you see why this doesn't make sense?

Your first "official" selfish act is to adopt this program. I want you to work it with intensity *and* consider that you are staging your own, personal intervention.

Changing Your Belief System

According to Martin Fishbein, Ph.D. and Distinguished Professor at the University of Pennsylvania (which happens to be my alma mater), "The study of health behavior is really a way to determine

> **What do they tell you on an airplane when the oxygen masks come down in the event of a change in pressure?** Put your mask on first; then help your children and the elderly. Why? Because in that way, you are strong enough to take charge and take care of those in need. Our instinct is not to do that, even though we have been told repeatedly to do so. We think we should help everyone else first, while desperately gasping for air and possibly passing out. But once you are toast, who is going to be there to help the others? Do you see this flawed belief system? Ask yourself if you would put on your own oxygen mask first? If your answer is "no," let's work on making that a "yes."

how to design interventions that change or reinforce beliefs." I like that approach a lot. Let's face it: changing your belief system does require an intervention similar to what we see on television or in movies when people "stage" an intervention for alcohol or drug abuse. Drug addicts and alcoholics believe they are really okay, that they don't really have a problem.[1] You may be thinking: "But alcohol and drug addition is a disease." Ah, that's a great point. In fact, researchers at Tufts University are looking into whether food addiction is truly an addiction and their preliminary research indicates that the answer is yes. Overeating is also a disease—and one that happens to be extremely contagious. I will cover that in chapter 9, as I urge you to look at the potential "obesogenic" environment in which you live and work, and the people with whom you live and work. Food addiction is a function of both the mind and the body. Your body is not meant to be overweight.

You've trained it to be that way and made it accustomed to asking for more food. You may also have trained your brain to behave the way it does around the whole subject of food, especially an unhealthy combination of salt, sugar, and fat. If you are struggling with your weight, and have been for a while, you need to start owning your behavior and not making excuses. Owning bad dietary behavior is the first step to changing your belief system. Once you change your belief system, I will give you a plan to follow that proves that you can lose weight without starving or excessively exercising.

How can I help you believe—really *believe*—that selfish is good? That will occur the moment you begin this plan, as the following changes begin to occur:

1. You will immediately start to lose weight. Seeing the scale go down will inspire you. Yes, you *are* going to get on the scale. But I will be there with you, spiritually holding your hand as you take those two big steps to success—on the scale each day.

2. Your clothes will instantly start to fit better, since you are embarking upon an exercise program that blasts off the inches faster than ever before. That's the recomposition I was telling you about in the introduction. You will very quickly feel leaner and sexier and—trust me—both selfish *and* sexy is good!

3. Your energy levels will soar, since you will be taking much better care of both your mind and your body. Energy levels also soar as you lose weight, since everything you do on a daily basis becomes that much easier. I believe energy levels are like bank accounts in which you make deposits and withdrawals. The more I teach you how to deposit more energy and make smaller withdrawals, the more your energy levels will explode.

Why People Fail

Why is this especially important for Petites? Well, as you will see in the next chapter when we work the numbers, you need to be committed for this plan to work and to work the plan so that you don't end up last on your list. As a Petite, you have a limited margin for error, but don't be discouraged by that. As I said in the introduction, you have probably been on plans that didn't work because they were more suitable for taller women and didn't speak directly to you. This program will work—in just twenty-one days!

Here is a statistic that may shock you: 97 percent of all people who attempt weight loss regain all the weight (and then some) in a five-year period. Now, before you get discouraged, I want you to understand that my personal success rate is around 75 percent. That's right, 75 percent of the people I have personally coached, or who have worked with my team of trainers, or who have followed the programs outlined in my past books have lost weight and *kept it off.* I know this to be true because the vast majority of them are in regular contact with me. But I've been in this business for decades. There are very few competitive authors or doctors or trainers or dietitians who can claim that much experience or that consistent a success rate. There are also very few comparable professionals who have worked one-on-one with as many people as I have over the years. It's that direct contact that makes the difference and, through trial and error, this has led to this winning program. I've helped thousands of petite women slim down and stay slim and I will do the same for you.

And I know why I succeed where so many fail. Because I provide a comprehensive plan and don't just deal with one variable, like what you eat. To promise weight loss by changing one variable alone (like eliminating carbs, which hasn't worked) is a sham and a waste of your time. In this book, I give you *everything* you need to achieve success.

Most people have only a 3 percent chance of success because:

- They tried a gimmick (Tai Bo—*please!*) that didn't work, got discouraged, and then went back to their old belief system and behaviors and proceeded to gain even more weight.

- They lost a few pounds by changing one variable (this time, they stopped eating by 7:00 P.M.—*wrong!*), then resumed their old belief system and behaviors as soon as they were "done" with their weight-loss plan. They subsequently gained all the weight back and then some.

No More Excuses

I wrote my second book, *Flip the Switch*, because so many readers wrote to me and said, "I love the concepts in your book but I just can't get started." They then listed excuses, and the beliefs that accompanied them:

- I have bad genes.

- I have a slow metabolism.

- I don't have the time.

- I can't get the energy.

- I *hate* to exercise.

- I *love* to eat.

- I'm a woman (yes, they actually used that as an excuse).

- It's just too late for me to even try.

These readers were passionately holding on to what kept them overweight and, in many instances, gaining weight. But by educating my readers and proving to them that they would lose weight (which is what will happen to you), I created the necessary shift in their belief system that translated into far better results-producing behavior.

For a moment, let me address the last bullet point above: "It's just too late for me to even try." Petites, it's *never* too late. You can start, right now, to make a shift in your body weight, your body's composition, your posture, your energy levels, the aging process, you name it. All you have to do is follow this plan, trust me, and truly believe that it will work. I've even helped Petites in their eighties get into far better shape, lose weight, and live a pain-free life. The wear and tear on your joints from excess weight is not something I can repair, but I can take pressure off those joints by strengthening the muscles, the tendons that connect muscles to bones, and the ligaments that connect bones to other bones. That "support team" eases the pain and, in many instances, eliminates it. If you are a Petite, odds are that you have a mother or sister or children who are also Petites. Please don't ever feel that it's just too late. It's not.

I was very fortunate that my first book, *The Business Plan for the Body*, came out exactly when Diane Sawyer went public with her twenty-five-pound weight loss. She achieved this dramatic result by following my plan, exactly as it was outlined in that book. Diane told the world on *Good Morning America* that, not only did she lose weight, but she experienced her first "recomposition." She even showed provocative before-and-after pictures, demonstrating the results, which were very impressive. The plan took a lot of inches off her body, which truly shocked her. She had to buy a whole new wardrobe. Her arms alone each lost four inches. Think about that—four inches from each arm. Once again, she was proudly sporting sleeveless tops. Her hips and glutes also shrank, just as they did for Gayle King, Oprah's BFF. Gayle got with my program because the magazine profiled Diane's success, then put four other women to the test—one in her twenties, one in her thirties, one in her forties (Gayle), and one in her fifties. Gayle became my second "celebrity" success story. The participant in her thirties, Cindy Paragallo, is a Petite. She shrank noticeably, losing eleven pounds of fat. To this day, she looks great and just had her second child.

Since then, I have been fine-tuning my techniques, as there is tremendous new research available—some of which I will share—that proves that there is a right way and a wrong way to lose weight, especially for Petites. As a Petite, you need to embrace the fact that your size can and *should* be used to your advantage, and I will make sure that every inch of your body is sleek, slender, and sexy.

The Seven Behaviors of Successful Weight Loss

I have been perfecting this plan for years. In the process, I stumbled across some research that virtually mirrors my approach to weight loss. This study comes from the National Weight Control Registry, which looked at the common factors in people who have lost more than thirty pounds and have kept it off longer than three years. Here are the top seven factors, which I call the Seven Behaviors of Successful Weight Loss.[2]

1. Eat a low-fat diet. Only 23 percent of total calories should come from fat. That's really not hard at all, once you eliminate a few extremely high-fat foods. And you also must differentiate

between the good fats and the bad fats. I'm a huge fan of the good fats, and will actually give you even a touch more than 23 percent of your calories from fat. On my plan, you will be eating 25 percent of your calories from the right fats. Remember: selfish is good. Well so is fat—the "good" fat, that is. Consuming more fat helps keep satiety mechanisms high and hunger low.

2. Eat a low-calorie diet. Successful average-size dieters consume between 1300 and 1500 calories each day. As a Petite, you must eat fewer calories—at times. You will soon learn that there is a surprising twist to my eating plan. Sometimes, you will get many more calories. Plus, you will not feel hunger with my plan, which is what frightens most people away from low-calorie diets. On my plan, eating a low-calorie diet is results-producing, satisfying, and sustainable over time. That's the way you achieve long-lasting results!

3. Eat breakfast and control portion size. Breakfast is a *must* on this plan and all portions need to be sized for Petites. If you are regularly skipping breakfast, please promise me that you won't *ever* do that again. I mean it. Don't do it, unless you are dying to gain weight. Breakfast is the "jump start" to your metabolism and the trigger for "satiety." FYI, if you are skipping breakfast *and* exercising first thing in the morning on an empty stomach, then you are effectively telling your body both to starve *and* to stay fat. That's not the goal.

4. Get sixty to ninety minutes of physical activity per day. Don't think of this specifically as "exercise," which I will define in chapter 8, but rather as daily movement that comes from cleaning the house, commuting to work, gardening, walking to the bus or the car or a meeting, shopping, cooking, or standing while talking on the phone. This sixty-to-ninety-minute goal

may seem daunting, but you will be surprised at how quickly your everyday activities can add up. I will share my tricks in chapter 8, but right now, if you stand up and read this book for a few minutes, you are helping your body. If you walk around and read, you help it even more. Movement is essential. But this is not exercise; this is simply adding more daily movement to your life without making it a big issue.

5. Weigh in regularly. You must weigh in a minimum of once a week, although the research shows that daily weighing is even more effective. The belief that the scale doesn't matter is so very wrong. The scale is essential to long-term success. Don't be afraid of the scale. Embrace it! It's your second, new BFF— right after my exercise program. You must weight in at least once a week, but to really work the plan and accelerate results, I urge you to get on the scale every day. It just shows you how your body is adjusting to the plan and also gives you valuable data regarding three important indicators:

• **Your water balance.** If your weight is truly bouncing around by more than a pound or two, then you are causing water retention. Look at the foods you are eating and the liquids you are drinking to find the culprit, as I want you to banish water bloat for good. I will discuss this in the next chapter.

• **Your regularity.** Again, I talk about this in the next chapter, but if you find that you frequently have regularity issues, you can correct them using my eating and drinking recommendations.

• **Your cycle.** I find that Petites get hit pretty hard with regard to water retention both during their monthly cycle and during ovulation. Still, get on the scale and change your mind-set to consider that as "data" not "failure."

6. Establish a support system. You *must* have a weight-loss buddy. I believe that your support system is as crucial to your success as your adherence to the actual plan. The people around you and the environments you are put in can make or break your success. I guarantee that they will help you succeed and I was truly surprised to see that research agrees.

7. Watch less than ten hours of television a week. I have to be honest and say that this blew me away. But the more I thought about it, the more I realized that many of the people I know who struggle with weight spend a good deal of time sitting. Now, the research on sitting and weight gain is pretty compelling. We will address this later on. Just know that limiting your "recreational" sitting is a must, especially if you have to sit during most of the day at work or at your desk at home. Also, look at the time you spend in the car. Many classic "soccer moms" spend hours each day in the car. I know that I sometimes spend all day Saturday just chauffeuring my kids between gymnastics training, theater rehearsal, playdates, grocery shopping, errands, etc. I plan my day so that I am on foot as much as possible; if that isn't possible, I make sure that I hit the exercise hard in the morning and don't allow myself to sit and watch TV later in the day. Instead, I write, read, or watch TV in the kitchen, standing up.

I will reference these seven behaviors repeatedly throughout this book, with the goal of changing your belief system regarding each one of them. Take, for example, the need to weigh in regularly. At my main studio in Chicago, we ask our staff to weigh each client *at least* once a week, although we actually prefer that it happen more often, even every session. The clients who agree to this practice generally lose weight. Those who refuse are not "losers" in a positive sense. They avoid the scale—no, they flatly refuse to get on the scale—and by doing so, they avoid the reality and hold on to their belief that they don't need to weigh in to lose weight. Excuse me, but yes you do! You have conducted your own, personal research study that proves that, if you don't regularly get on the scale, you won't lose weight. Better yet, if you don't regularly get on the scale, you will probably gain weight!

I am very committed when it comes to getting results. By getting on the scale, you hold *yourself* accountable, since I can't personally be there. You think that you are working my plan. Then you get on the scale and it doesn't agree with you. The scale is your "data." It is what gives you the "red flag" you need to examine where you are straying from the program. Are you really sticking with the eating plan as it's laid out? Are you really hitting your exercise with the intensity required? Are you truly sleeping seven to eight hours each night? The scale holds you accountable for success and non-success. When you don't lose weight, you are forced to reassess your commitment and behavior. Without the scale, you can live in denial, which you may have done in the past. That's why it's your second BFF. (I have a secret strategy to hold you accountable to your daily weigh-ins that I will share with you in chapter 9—an easy technique that can have an enormous impact on your results.)

Let me give you another example. I am a resource speaker for Vistage International, the largest CEO think tank in the world. I travel all over the world presenting to these CEOs, many of whom are entrepreneurs and highly educated, successful people. When I ask the members to describe their goals for health, weight, and energy levels, with virtually 95 percent consistency the breakfast-skippers struggle with weight. The reason I bring up this point is that, even with the research that I will share with you in chapter 2, which finds that breakfast is essential for weight loss, their *belief* systems remain intact with excuses like "I'm too busy," or "I'm not hungry." They aren't willing to change, even when presented with

> **Hunger only for breakfast.** *The only time you should feel hunger is first thing in the morning, after you have fasted for eight or more hours, depending on how long you slept and if you ate something close to bedtime. If you continually skip breakfast, your body just stops asking for it and you don't feel hungry. Once you start eating breakfast every single day (I don't want you to skip even one), you will feel hungry each morning but far less hungry later in the day. It's simply another example of how your belief that you don't need to eat breakfast translates into your behavior. You decide that you are not going to eat breakfast, and your body follows the wrong message. Eat breakfast—please!*

overwhelming proof that breakfast and weight loss go hand in hand. It's baffling how these highly educated people, who rely upon research, facts, and numbers, refuse to change.

If there is one of the seven behaviors listed above that you have already identified as problematic, then I urge you to start working on adjusting your belief system in that area *now*. Don't wait. If you can identify your biggest stumbling block first, you will then have more time to devote to the necessary changes.

This is imperative for you as a Petite, because you do not possess the same margin for error that taller women do. Your body requires fewer calories each day and must possess a productive, high-powered metabolism. Each of these factors is proven to result in weight loss and must be honored. I can't make you change the behavior required if I can't change that stubborn belief system that disagrees with and ultimately sabotages your chance of success.

Taking Control

From this page forward, I want this to be your mantra:

- My belief system has been flawed. I now believe that selfish is good!

- My new belief system will lead to new behaviors that reinforce placing myself first.

- My new beliefs and behaviors will make me much more energetic, productive, and calm. My stress levels will diminish and that will benefit everyone around me, because I made the decision to place myself first.

- My new beliefs will enable me to lose weight and keep it off!

Just saying these things will make you feel better and, with repetition, you will really start to *believe* them and *live* them.

It's a bit like believing you can "live your best life," which has been Oprah's message for years. Only with that belief intact can you actually start to "live your best life."

Your homework, starting today, is to plan just five minutes to focus on yourself. In those five, pre-determined minutes—yes, *plan* them—I want you to:

1. Think about what you are going to eat for the rest of the day and tomorrow.

2. Plan when you are going to exercise in the coming week. You just need three thirty-one-minute chunks, so that's not asking for a lot of time.

3. Eliminate one unnecessary task from your day. No, that basement closet does *not* need to be cleaned out today. Instead,

make a cup of tea, because tea boosts your metabolism and helps you lose weight. Isn't that what this book is supposed to be about?

4. Breathe. I give you a stress-relieving breathing exercise on pages 267–268. Peek at it now if you feel you need it.

I'm only asking for five minutes. Clearly, you have that time to give to yourself—because you now believe that selfish is good!

CHAPTER 2

METABOLISM
Your "Weapon of Mass Reduction"

Metabolism: the set of chemical reactions that occur in living organisms to maintain life. FYI, these *chemical reactions* burn lots and lots of *calories*.

Effective, permanent weight loss is all about an optimized, "calorie burning" metabolism, which is why I call it your "weapon of mass reduction."

Stop and think for a moment. Why have you not succeeded at weight loss in the past? No, don't think. I have the answer. You were not a success at weight loss because virtually all the diets you have been on in the past totally destroyed your metabolism.

Quick. Go turn your blender, fan, or hair dryer on high. Think of that as many, many calories being spent (which is good) at the highest possible speed. Now turn it on medium. Ah, not quite the energy (calories) that was blasting before. It's slower. Finally, turn it on low. Now it's humming along in comparison to the two other settings. That is the metabolic consequence of 99.99 percent of all diets you have followed in the past. You turned your motor from high to low—and, in the process, you gained all the weight back and then some, and wondered why. You may even have berated yourself and called yourself a failure. I refer to "failure" as the "F word"; I prefer to call it "non-success," or just NS. I am here to tell you that you have destroyed your metabolism by decreasing your precious metabolism-boosting tissue—*muscle*. But before you panic, rest assured that I will show you how to fix that.

Here is the reason you and virtually every other woman who has gone on a diet has failed:

Diet for Weight Loss = Diminished Lean Muscle

When you lose weight on virtually all diets, you lose approximately 60 to 70 percent fat and 30 to 40 percent muscle. That's a disaster because:

Diminished Lean Muscle = Diminished Metabolism

Another way to put that is:

Lean Muscle Down = Metabolism Down

That's the NS formula.

In this program, the *success* equation for Petites is:

Lean Muscle Up = Metabolism Up

Without a high-performing metabolism, you are doomed to fail at weight loss because your body will burn very few calories on a daily basis. And that means you need to eat even *fewer* calories in order to lose weight, which is all but impossible. You're living on "low."

Many women hear the word "muscle" and run for the hills. *They have this vision of pumped up, steroid-ridden, "freaky-looking" women who ungracefully "grace" the cover of women's body-builder magazines. That is not the visual we are looking for. If you don't believe me, Google Petra Nemcova, the 2004 cover model of* Sports Illustrated's *swimsuit edition, who just last spring was on* Dancing with the Stars. *She is magnificent. A few years ago, she and I did a television show together regarding the secrets of celebrity fitness. Guess what Petra does all the time. Strength training to maintain her muscle and blast off her fat. Is she lean, long, sexy, and gorgeous? Google the pictures of her and you be the judge.*

Come on, you've tried the NS formula in the past. Why not do it the right way this time, since you already know that it didn't work the other way.

When I say this to 99.9 percent of dieters, who admit to me that they are NS at losing weight, they say, "but I loved that diet." Can you believe it? They love something that brought them failure and then they defend it! Talk about a deeply, painfully flawed belief system.

Isn't Einstein's definition of insanity doing the same thing over and over again and expecting a different result? Why would anyone embrace the same *results-free* strategy over and over and expect a different outcome? They do so because their *belief* system is so very out of whack.

So let's get to the heart of that often misunderstood word, "metabolism."

Understanding Your Basal Metabolic Rate

Each of us possesses a basal metabolic rate, or BMR, defined as:

The amount of energy expended while at rest in a neutrally temperate environment, in the post-absorptive state (meaning that the digestive system is inactive, which requires about twelve hours of fasting in humans). The release of energy in this state is sufficient only for the functioning of the vital organs, such as the heart, lungs, brain and the rest of the nervous system, liver, kidneys, sex organs, muscles and skin. BMR decreases with age and with the loss of lean body mass. Increasing muscle mass increases BMR. [1]

Please note the last two sentences of this definition: BMR decreases with age and with the loss of lean body mass. Increasing lean muscle mass increases BMR. My eating and exercise plan will keep your BMR from going down, even as you age. I know for a fact that the metabolic rate of some senior Petites I've worked with went up, because they started saying to me things like: "Jim, you know I have to have my hair colored every three weeks instead of every four. The roots seem to be showing faster as my stylist tells me my hair is growing faster." That alone, along with nail growth (another easy indicator), can prove that your metabolism is accelerating.

As a Petite, your goal is to do *everything* in your power to maintain and increase your metabolism, *especially* when you diet or restrict calories. When restricting calories, your body senses that there is not a readily available source of food. So the very smart human body slows down its need for food or calories. How does your body go about slowing itself down? It atrophies one of the body's most metabolically active tissues—muscle. Muscle burns between twenty-two and thirty-six calories per pound per day. That is why it is so very important to your metabolism. If you diminish your muscle tissue, which is what happens when you diet without exercise or skip breakfast, your metabolism will go down. Again, less muscle will lead to a slower metabolism. You *never* want that to happen. By following my eating and exercise plan, you can prevent that from happening.

For years, I have heard countless excuses concerning metabolism. I must be perfectly clear that the majority of them are unfounded, because virtually 99 percent of the time, the problem is not your metabolism. The problem is your behavior. No, actually it's your belief system (like believing that cardio is the key to weight loss, which it is not) that led to your behavior (like performing cardio, a great weight-*gain* program). Sorry to be blunt, but it's the truth. Stop for a moment and think:

- Were you always this weight?

- Was there a time when you were at a lower weight?

- Did this weight just creep up one pound at a time?

- Did you weigh yourself often to stop the increase?

- Did you count calories?

- Did you exercise the right way or did you perform cardio?

- Are you getting enough sleep?

- Are you stressed to the max?

How, then, can you blame your metabolism? I bet your metabolism rocks. Or at least it used to rock before you annihilated it with a diet. But I can help you fix that! Don't beat yourself up about the past. It's over. Let's move forward, with me as your guide, and shed that fat once and for all.

Recently, there was a picture in a magazine of Oak Street Beach in Chicago, my hometown. The picture was from the 1950s and everyone in it looked as if they had stepped out of a beach movie from exactly that era. Everyone was lean and I mean really lean. There was not an overweight or obese person in sight. Now, fast-forward to today. I am frequently on that beach with my kids, and the vast majority of men and women are much bigger, and I don't mean by just a few pounds. Do you think our genes mutated in a few decades? *No.* It's *impossible.* Our behavior mutated—big-time—so please don't blame your genes. Instead, let's get to work on optimizing your metabolism through new beliefs and behaviors.

Optimizing Your Metabolism

What healthy factors do affect metabolism? Don't get me started on diet pills and smoking, which, yes, do boost metabolism, but do it in a very dangerous way. Is smelling like an ashtray and/or dying really worth it? Can you really do anything to increase your metabolism? The answer to that question is a big *yes.* Here are some of the issues that you can address to optimize your metabolism.

Thyroid

If you are feeling low in energy, depressed or anxious, have thinning hair and brittle nails, or have issues with constipation, irregular menstrual cycle, infertility, or low sex drive, you may be suffering from hypothyroid (too little thyroid). Now, many women I know claim that the reason for their weight gain is a slow thyroid, but a very small percentage of these women actually have the dysfunction. Once again, it's your behavior that is problematic, not your thyroid.

If you suffer from either hypothyroid (too slow) or hyperthyroid (too fast, which is also not good for your health), then properly balancing your thyroid through medication is essential to an optimized metabolism for weight loss. Have your levels checked regularly by your doctor and be vigilant about taking your medication. Also, don't wait if you feel there is a problem. Get on the phone, make the appointment, and get in to see your doctor if necessary. If your primary care physician is not giving you the attention or answering all your questions, then go to a specialist. There is no reason to live even one day with thyroid dysfunction, especially if you've already been diagnosed. Take your medication, as the percentage of people who don't take their medication or don't take it properly is enormous.

Digestion

Skipping meals is a *killer* to your metabolism, especially breakfast. Those who regularly skip breakfast have a 450 percent greater chance of being overweight or obese.[2] Some research has shown that regular breakfast-skippers possess metabolisms that are diminished by as much as 5 to 10 percent. British researchers even found that "breakfast size was inversely related to waist size," meaning the bigger the breakfast, the smaller the waist. Those are compelling reasons to eat breakfast.

I want you to eat immediately after you get up. I eat within fifteen minutes of getting up in the morning. It doesn't have to be an entire breakfast. Many times, I eat a piece or serving of fruit first, then exercise, then eat the rest a little later. Also note that for anyone exercising first thing if the morning, you must eat first or you risk burning muscle. Eat approximately 100 calories before you exercise—such as a piece of fruit, a yogurt, or a piece of

100-calorie whole-wheat toast—then eat the rest of your breakfast right after. This should contain more protein.

Muscle

If you regularly skip breakfast to cut calories and lose weight, you're in good company with the likes of Diane Sawyer. She used to do it before she worked with me, and so did other celebs and soccer moms I've helped in the past. Again, when you skip meals, your body believes there is not a readily available source of fuel. But you should never tell your body that there is a scarcity of food, as it will do everything in its power to slow your metabolism to prolong your life. This is a classic example of your beliefs affecting your behavior, which directly affects your metabolism. Don't tell me that you have a bad metabolism before asking yourself: "What am I doing to slow my metabolism? Am I holding myself accountable for my beliefs and behaviors?"

The way your body slows your metabolism is to break down muscle. That's right; your body goes right to the muscle because it is so metabolically active. It reduces your muscle mass in order to keep you alive. It's exactly like whacking off one of the blades of a fan. Suddenly, even when turning at the same speed, the fan moves less air. But your body only breaks down muscle because you told it to. It was not the body's desire to do that. Your *belief system* told you that you didn't need or want to eat breakfast. This led to damaging *behavior*—not eating breakfast—which resulted in the outcome—you made your muscle and your metabolism go bye-bye.

Satiety

Satiety mechanisms are highest in the morning. Therefore, what you eat in the morning will actually determine how hungry you are later in the day. That's the reason behind the research that showed an "inverse" relationship between breakfast and your waist. If your satiety mechanisms are firing at full throttle in the morning, then you will get more "bang for your buck" by eating more breakfast. It's like fueling a fire. When it's blazing and you throw on another log, that log quickly ignites and keeps the fire burning strong *and* long. That "ignition" is the response of your satiety mechanisms when you eat more breakfast. Later in the day, you are far less hungry. And be honest. Isn't it later in the day and into the evening when you really get into trouble with your food choices? By the way, the latest class of diet drugs is tailored to increase a feeling of fullness (satiety), but they are known to have substantial side effects. Eat a substantial breakfast and skip the drugs *and* the side effects.

Think about it for a moment. Many of you have to get up early, around 6:00 A.M. If you eat breakfast, you may not be hungry again until noon; that's six hours later. Then, around 4:00, you get "the munchies" and are rooting around for a snack. That's four hours from lunch. Then around 6:30, just two and a half hours later, you're hungry for dinner, and by 8:00, just an hour and a half later, you're back at the munchies.

Eating a much more substantial breakfast at 6:00 A.M. will result in you not being nearly as hungry later in the day and probably not hungry at all. Why? Satiety. You simply feel full throughout the day (actually for about twenty-four hours) when you "front load," or eat a bigger breakfast and allocate more of your calories to much earlier in the day. Eat breakfast and you will physically need to eat less *later* in the day and at night. The old adage, "eat like a king for breakfast, like a prince for lunch, and like a pauper for dinner" is absolutely right.

You can control your metabolism by how you behave—how and when you eat, exercise, sleep, stress out, etc. Just skipping breakfast, or any meal for that matter, will weaken your metabolism. *Don't do it!* Even when I drill this into some of my clients, readers, and followers, they still continue to do it. Come on. The excuse that you don't have time doesn't fly with me, as I know it takes less than a minute to eat a hard-boiled egg, scoop down a container of low-fat yogurt with fruit, or drink a well-balanced protein shake. Remember, the excuse that you're not hungry also doesn't fly, because the only reason you are not hungry in the morning is that your body is tired of asking for food. It just gives up trying and you subsequently don't feel hungry anymore. You blew out your body's hunger mechanisms. But you can reverse that by eating breakfast—a key to my plan. To be perfectly honest, the only time you should feel hungry is first thing in the morning. My goal for the rest of the day is to keep hunger at bay. If you still don't plan to eat breakfast (there's that flawed belief system again), then you are destined to stay at your present weight—and then some.

Body Weight

In the next chapter, I will introduce you to the Harris Benedict Equation. If you are at a heavier body weight, your BMR goes up. For the overweight, the excuse of having a bad metabolism is generally inaccurate. You actually have a higher metabolism than you would at a lighter weight, because everything you do—from getting out of a chair to shopping to running to your office to cleaning—takes more energy since there is *more* of you to move around.

The obese tend to expend more energy than lean people of comparable height, sex, and bone structure, which means their metabolisms are typically burning off *more* calories rather than fewer.[3]

In addition, for the overweight, digesting all those extra calories actually boosts their metabolism. Their bodies have to work harder to digest all the additional calories. I've told you that your body slows down when you restrict calories, which is what you have to do to lose weight. The exact opposite happens when you overeat. Your body actually speeds up, as it wants to burn off some of the calories rather than store them as fat. The problem is that you may overeat so many calories that your body can't speed up to that degree, so you gain weight. Please own this fact and stop making excuses that don't help you achieve weight loss. And if you have annihilated your metabolism with repeated, gimmicky diets, I can still help you fix that, so don't blame your metabolism. Blame your past behavior, which you can change starting today.

Spicy Food

Did you ever wonder why you start sweating when you eat food with some added "kick." Well, like a fever—which is also a boost in your metabolism as your very smart body attacks the infection or whatever foreign substance has entered it—your body speeds up when you eat spicy food and that translates into a bump in your metabolism. Some new research out of Canada even proves that spice in food may also help to tip satiety mechanisms. This new research took adult men and served one group an appetizer with hot sauce and another group without. If you can believe it, the group that consumed the hot sauce ate, on average, 200 fewer calories at lunch and later in the day. Capsaicin, a compound found in chili peppers, was what they used to spice up the appetizers and the researchers theorize that it may work as an appetite suppressant.[4] I have always found that moderately spicy food also tastes better. One of my favorites is lemon pepper, which is recommended as a spice in your eating plan. I avoid the salt shaker for obvious reasons, but that does not mean that your food can't be tasty and low in calories.

Moreover, spices are packed with antioxidants. In the January 2010 issue of *Nutrition Journal*, researchers claimed that "culinary herbs and spices have the highest antioxidant content of all foods."[5] Therefore, you receive *überbenefits* from spices, including enhanced health. In fact, some research says that combining spices makes them even more potent. Spices can give you a metabolic kick, as all spices—especially capsaicin, black pepper, and ginger—give your metabolism an extra jump start. And even small increases in calorie burn can add up to big results over time. When you see your eating plan in chapter 5, you will see that spices play a starring role, for all these reasons.

Caffeine

In chapter 7, I will tell you all about the true magic of tea and, to some extent, coffee. Yes, it does boost your metabolism, but you need to use it intelligently and cautiously.

Lean Muscle Tissue

Ah, the mother lode when it comes to an optimized metabolism! But you have to wait until chapter 8 to hear about that, or you can flip there now to find out why your lean muscle tissue is the motor of your metabolism and the magic bullet when it comes to a metabolism that gets the weight off and then keeps it off.

The Fidget Factor

Mayo Clinic researchers outfitted lean and obese individuals with underwear with sensors that monitored their every movement. What they found was that the overweight people simply moved *less* than the leaner participants. I have always been a fan of this research. For years, I've noticed that overweight people sit a lot, while those that are lean move around more. Now, to be clear, I don't know which came first, the weight or the lack of movement. Of course, overweight people have told me for years that they are not comfortable moving around a lot, giving a number of reasons—it is simply difficult for them, or it is painful for joints (especially knees and hips) to bear the added weight, or they are most likely not living in an environment where anyone is moving around much. When was the last time you saw an obese family on the front lawn playing touch football, riding bikes, or playing tennis?

I even ask spouses, partners, family members, or co-workers what they observe when it comes to activity levels. Hands down, I hear comments like "He or she is always moving around" when referring to the lean and, conversely, "He or she just sits around the house" for those *less* lean.

Researchers theorize that part of this may be genetic (albeit, a small part), but yes, you can program yourself to get off the couch if inactivity has become your habit. In addition to what is defined as "exercise," I still do, personally, move around constantly and urge you to do the same.

Very recently, research came out about the dangers of sitting for many hours in the day. This relates to one of the Seven Behaviors of Successful Weight Loss—watching less than ten hours of television a week. The findings went so far as to say that, even if you exercise for thirty minutes a day, eight hours of sitting cancels out all the benefits of those thirty minutes.[6] Yikes! There's a good reason to start a "stand up and lose" movement in this country!

I walk around when I talk on the phone, at home or at the office. I try to stand up (which is what I am doing right now as I work on this chapter) and put my laptop on a kitchen counter in my home or on a counter at the office. There is also research that shows that you are more creative when you are moving, since more blood is flowing to your brain. Looks like standing up is a "win-win" proposition for more than just weight loss.

Now, I find that recommendations like "park your car at the farthest space and walk" are highly impractical, as my clients rarely subscribe to these behaviors. So I needed to create certain rules that may make more sense to you. Here, just to give you an example, are some of my movement habits while traveling, when I know I will be sitting for a period of time:

1. No moveable walkways, escalators, or elevators. I walk and climb, and that also makes you think twice when packing, since you have to pick up your suitcase (even if it rolls) from time to time. And if you do use the moveable walkway, then please, *walk*. It's not a moveable "standway"! Don't just stand there—move!

2. If my flight is delayed, I take to the concourse and walk and talk, as I am generally on my cell phone (but with my Bluetooth or other earpiece, as I do believe too much cell phone use can be hazardous).

3. When in the air, I purposely get up to go to the bathroom when there is a line. That way, I get to stand up without being harassed by the flight attendant.

As a Petite, you need a calorie-blasting metabolism to get the weight off, because it's harder for you to create a caloric deficit. Don't forget that you have to expend more calories than you take in to force your body to use its own stored energy source—fat! You will have a clearer understanding of this issue once you get through the next chapter and understand The Math of weight loss.

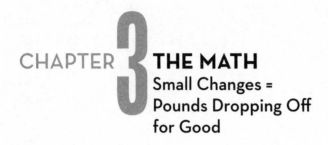

CHAPTER **3** **THE MATH**
Small Changes =
Pounds Dropping Off
for Good

You now understand that a booming metabolism translates to a smaller, sexier, "tighter-lighter" physique (I will explain why the quotes are around "tighter-lighter" later). Now, let's go to the next step—understanding simple math. The math we are concerned with here applies to women of all shapes, heights, and sizes, but is especially important to Petites.

As with most math problems, we start with an equation. The classic equation that determines your body weight is:

Calories In (Food) – Calories Out (Activity and Metabolism) = Your Present Body Weight

Most people are shocked when I tell them that their present body weight is the function of every single calorie they have ever consumed, minus every calorie burned through activity and metabolism. This covers your *entire* life. Instead of embracing the power of this equation, most people hold on to certain beliefs that they feel are the reason for their present body weight. In fact, it just comes back to The Math each time you lose weight (that's good), or gain weight (that's not so good), or stay the same (which may or may not be good, depending on the number).

You should also realize that if you are carrying extra weight and the scale is staying within a small range (say two to three pounds), then your equation is in balance. Your calories in are roughly equal to your calories out. Now, you may not be happy with this number and want to reduce it, which is probably why you have this book in your hands. But I need you to own up to the fact that *you* have balanced your equation to determine your present weight. Once I teach you how to manipulate the equation, you will have the knowledge to bring that number down.

In this chapter, we will look at the simple numbers for weight loss. In subsequent chapters, we will dig deeper into other factors that influence this weight-loss equation—factors like what foods positively influence your equation, what habits positively influence your equation, what activities enhance your weight loss, and what exercise is essential to your weight loss. But for now, let's think of this as Weight-Loss Math 101.

Petite Math

You may be wondering why this equation is so specifically important to Petites. It is because smaller figures do not possess a very large margin for error. Once you embrace the numbers and understand their importance to weight loss, you will, for the first time, understand why your prior weight-loss attempts did not succeed or only worked for a short (no pun intended) period of time.

Let me give you an example. Let's say you are the lifeguard at your community pool. There are actually two pools: one that is considered the "baby" pool, for children of a certain age, size, and ability level, and another much larger, Olympic-size pool that is used by the majority of people. At the end of each night, you have to refill both pools, and you do so by placing a hose in each one. By accident, you leave the water hoses turned on at the same pressure in each pool. What happens?

1. The baby pool fills up much faster, since it is smaller. Therefore, it overflows much more water and really soaks the area around it.

2. The Olympic pool fills up more slowly and doesn't overflow as much, since it takes a lot more water to fill it up given its size.

Petites are the baby pool. When you overeat, you fill up faster, just like the baby pool. And all that extra water soaking the surrounding area, for you, represents body fat.

Your taller counterparts also fill up—no doubt about that—but they don't get nearly the amount of overflow, which is why they gain less body fat (unless they really, really overeat).

The Weight-Loss Equation

Now, let's examine a few facts about this math that can help to convince you of its importance.

Fact 1: Your body weight, right now, is the function of this equation:

Calories In – Calories Out = Your Present Body Weight

Now, take that equation one step further.

Calories In (Food and Drink) – Calories Out (Activity and Metabolism) = Your Present Body Weight

I am going to help you manipulate this equation to bring your "calories in" down and your "calories out" up to create a caloric deficit that will bring your body weight down. In the past, you have created a caloric surplus, and that is why your weight is presently higher than you would like it to be. Surplus equals weight gain and deficit equals weight loss.

Fact 2: One pound = 3500 calories. This is often misunderstood. I frequently ask audiences how many calories equal one pound and, if you can believe it, I have received answers as low as 50 and as high as 50,000! Clearly, there is some confusion. A calorie, for the record, is a unit of energy. Your goal is to balance your equation, "energy in minus energy out," which I further define as, "calories in minus calories out."

In the very recent past, some bestselling books have rejected this equation, referring to research that says it's much more about the quality of calories you consume than the quantity. They disagree with the body-weight equation above, which I clearly embrace. I want to be perfectly clear. I *know* this equation works, as I have been relying on it for myself, my staff, my clients, and my readers for years. In the next chapter, we'll talk about the quality of food, as there are foods I want you to embrace and foods I want you to eliminate or reduce in your daily diet. But I simply cannot agree that this body-weight equation is without value. It is the starting point for any successful weight-loss plan. If my theory of "calories in minus calories out" didn't work, it stands to reason that I wouldn't have the voice I have in this industry. Nor would I have everyone from celebrities to CEOs to soccer moms clamoring for my advice and proven results. Sorry to sound a bit "full of myself," but I've been in this weight-loss business for over twenty-five years, working directly with clients. Many of the people who denounce this equation have never actually worked with a single person who has successfully lost weight. I have, thousands of times!

If you are presently struggling with your weight and not happy with what the scale reports (and you should be weighing yourself every day), then I need to help you rebalance your equation. Here is how I want you to look at weight gain and calories in the future:

- If you gain a pound, then you have consumed 3500 more calories than *your* present body required.

- If you gain five pounds, then you have consumed 3500 x 5 or 17,500 more calories than *your* present body required.

- If you gain ten pounds, then you have consumed 3500 x 10 or 35,000 more calories than *your* body required.

- If you are up fifty pounds, then you have consumed 175,000 more calories than *your* body required.

I hope you see how these numbers add up. The exact same thing happens as you lose weight. To take off one pound, you must create a deficit of 3500 calories and so on. It works in both directions.

Please take note of the fact that I've italicized *your* body. There can be slight (and I mean very slight) metabolic differences in women, even women of the same age, height, and weight. But please, stop comparing yourself to others. Just worry about *your* body and getting it to the healthier, leaner state that I *know* it was in at an earlier stage in your life.

Pregnancy and Weight Gain

Let's be honest—we all use some sort of excuse to justify our present weight. I think I have heard every conceivable excuse from my clients, friends, and followers over the years. It's human nature. I know I made excuses when I was overweight.

One common excuse used by women is that they are still holding on to "baby weight." This is a big one, regardless of how long ago you had your last baby. So many Petites have told me that their first pregnancy was the catalyst for their weight gain, which they are still struggling with today, years or perhaps decades later. What I find is that, outside of the obvious weight gain that occurred with the pregnancy and post-baby, your schedule totally changes. With the stresses of motherhood, exercise, low-calorie meals, and sleep are the first to go. Therefore, it really isn't just the baby weight that's responsible for your weight gain; it's really more your post-baby behavior and your new belief system. Look, I know from having two children (no, I didn't actually carry them) that it's tough with a newborn in the house and you are pressed for time and energy. But just understand, for the sake of your body weight, that had you gone back to your pre-baby beliefs and their accompanying behaviors—with your "calories in" lower and your "calories out" higher—your equation would have rebalanced and your current weight would be much closer to your pre-baby weight. Plus, you clearly need more energy to take care of your new baby and most likely a job, a husband, possibly other children, aging parents, you name it. When I get you leaner, I *guarantee* that you will get an energy boost. And don't get overwhelmed by the big picture—consider every pound you lose post-baby (regardless of the baby's age) to be a victory. Follow this plan and in no time, you will be at your goal.

Another frequent excuse for weight gain during pregnancy is that you are "eating for two." Ready for the reality? Most women are shocked to hear that, when pregnant, you get to eat approximately 300 additional calories a day. No, that is not a typo. You truly should only be eating around 300 extra calories a day—two pieces of fruit (100 calories each) and a yogurt (many are right around 100 calories) or two eggs (around 90 to 100 calories each)

> ***If you are presently overweight and are pregnant***
> *or planning on becoming pregnant in the future, be very
> careful with pregnancy weight gain. Address this issue
> with your doctor, as I don't claim to be one, but Dr. Raul
> Artal of St. Louis University School of Medicine says that
> pregnancy is one of the main causes of obesity in women.
> I strongly agree, as I've seen it and heard it numerous
> times from clients. He goes on to say that, in the past,
> there was a fear that not gaining enough weight would
> hurt the development of the fetus.[1] That opinion has now
> changed, as many women begin their pregnancies over-
> weight, which presents a different scenario and environ-
> ment in which the fetus grows. Researchers now believe
> that women who are already overweight should gain
> little (if any) weight at all, as it won't in any way harm the
> fetus. It may lead to a slightly lower birth weight, but may
> minimize other complications like gestational diabetes
> and high blood pressure whose risks may be greater than
> a lower birth weight for the baby.*

and piece of whole-wheat toast or Ezekiel bread (right around 100 calories). So many women I know gain a tremendous amount of weight because they believe that pregnancy means they have forty weeks of "Get Out of Jail Free" cards and can therefore eat with reckless abandon. I actually don't blame them, as that is the prevailing wisdom. And what makes it worse is all the pregnant women depicted on television and in the movies who do exactly that. Please know that it's not healthy for you or for your unborn baby. I know, as I have helped hundreds of women, especially Petites, carry healthy babies, have easier deliveries, develop fewer stretch marks (if any), and then bounce back to their pre-baby weight in no time. Many of them were in their late thirties or early forties when this occurred, so I'm not talking about the youngsters who frequently bounce back faster.

Calculating Your Basal Metabolic Rate

Another excuse I often here is "I have a bad or slow metabolism." There are, in fact, behaviors that can slow your metabolism, like skipping meals (especially breakfast) and eliminating exercise or exercising in the wrong way. But there are also behaviors that will rev your metabolism back up if it needs it and keep it revved up, even as you age. Keep in mind that your "calories out" number is a function of both your activity level and your metabolism. By increasing your metabolism, you can really accelerate your weight loss, since your metabolism burns many more calories than most activities and exercise because it burns calories around the clock. This is the way to get weight off that *stays* off, for good. It's also the weight that is *all* fat, and you have to love the idea of blasting fat off of your body!

Seventy-five percent of your metabolism is determined by your behavior. Only 25 percent is determined by your genes. You can only blame 25 percent of your present body weight on your metabolism, if any. You must take a closer look at your caloric intake, which leads me to the next excuse: I really don't eat that much. Since this chapter is all about The Math, let's examine this excuse using another equation.

Back in 2001, I introduced my readers to the Harris Benedict Equation, which is an approximation of how many calories your body presently requires to *stay* at your current weight. Our goal will be to use this equation to arrive at a lower body weight for you. While this is an approximation, I strongly believe it is a great way to illustrate The Math. I also like the fact that it not only gives you a greater understanding of what is going on with your present body weight, but is also a perfect starting point for losing the weight, fast.

Here is the actual equation, and I am only using the one that applies to women since, ladies, this book is for you. This calculation is available on the Internet, so don't get bogged down by the math. Just keep reading for now and plug the numbers in once you have finished this chapter.

Your Basal Metabolic Rate (BMR) = 655 + (4.35 x weight in pounds) + (4.7 x height in inches) - (4.7 x age in years)

Take the number that you calculate with the above equation and multiply it by the applicable activity multiplier listed below—and don't lie about your activity level! This level should reflect what you truly do on a daily basis now and not what you *aspire* to do in the future:

1. If you are sedentary (little or no exercise), multiply by 1.2.

2. If you are lightly active (some light exercise like walking or a sport one to three days a week), multiply by 1.375.

3. If you are moderately active (moderate exercise/sports like singles tennis three to five days a week), multiply by 1.55.

4. If you are very active (hard exercise/sports six to seven days a week), multiply by 1.725.

5. If you are extremely active (this is Olympic training, ladies, so probably does not apply to most of you), multiply by 1.9.

For the sake of illustration, let's say you are forty-two years old, 5'3" tall, and 170 pounds, and that you use lightly active as your multiplier. I am using these numbers because these were the starting numbers for the Petite client I referenced in the introduction who lost forty pounds (and to this day has kept it off) on this plan.

655 + (4.35 x 170 [weight]) + (4.7 x 63 [height in inches]) – (4.7 x 42 [age]) = 655 + 739.5 + 296.1 – 197.4 = 1493.2

1493.2 x (activity multiplier #2 or 1.375) = 2053.15

Therefore, my former client had to eat approximately 2053.15 calories a day to *maintain* her weight at that time. To lose just a pound a week (on my plan, you will easily lose three or four pounds a week during your first twenty-one days), she would have to eat 3500 fewer calories a week (because 3500 calories equals one pound). Remember, you have to create a caloric deficit to lose weight. Funny that 3500 is easily divisible by the seven days of the week. She would have to cut 500 calories a day (500 calories x 7 days = 3500 calories) to lose one pound. My client would have to have dropped her daily caloric intake to 1553.15 (2053.15 minus 500) to lose one pound a week. Again, please note, you will lose far more weight than that during your first twenty-one days on my plan, as you will also be shedding bloat, clearing out your intestines, *and* drastically enhancing your metabolism.

Weight loss is math, and you must understand that math if you truly want to succeed in the long run and not just for a short period of time.

The Yo-Yo Syndrome

Why do almost all the people you know who lose weight gain it all back? Once again, it's because of the math. Let's say that, in the example I just showed you, my client lost forty pounds, which is what she did lose. If her activity multiplier stayed the same, then her "after-weight-loss" equation looked like this:

655 + (4.35 x 130 [her new weight after losing 40 pounds]**) + (4.7 x 63** [clearly, her height had to stay the same]**) – (4.7 x 42** [her age stayed the same]**) = 655 + 565.5 + 296.1 – 197.4 = 1319.2**

1319.2 x 1.375 (the same activity multiplier as before) = 1813.9

If you recall, the calories originally required to maintain her weight at 170 pounds was 2053.15. Now, she only needs 1813.9 to maintain her weight at 130 pounds. While approximately 240 calories a day may not seem like a big deal, it could add up to a weight gain of twenty-five pounds a year—of fat! Not understanding this math is why such a huge percentage of people fail at weight loss. By doing the math, you can understand the adjustments that have to be made. Think about it this way. The smaller "baby" pool requires less water to fill up than the big pool. The same applies to you when you lose weight. After your weight loss, you will require fewer calories (although I will teach you some tricks that will enable you to eat more).

If the former client I am using throughout this example had been 5'9" instead of 5'3", she could have consumed 4.7 x 6 (the difference between being 5'9" and 5'3") and that would have given her an additional 28.2 calories each day. Take a look back at the equation and you will see what I am talking about if you are confused. Sounds like a small amount of calories, doesn't it? But what happens each year if this client eats like a woman who is 5'9"? She will gain approximately three pounds each and every year. That's thirty pounds a decade! That's ninety pounds after three decades! Does that sound at all like you and the way your weight has slowly

> *Sorry to be the bearer of bad news*—but for Petites, the numbers matter much more, since your height is a big factor in how many calories you require on a daily basis, whether you are gaining or losing or staying the same. I can't do anything about that, but that's the whole point of this book. I can work successfully with your height and get you results you desire.
>
> Again, this is one of the primary reasons so many of you have gained all your weight back (and then some) in the past. You didn't pay attention to The Math. Therefore, by returning to your previous calories (when you were at a higher weight), you created a caloric surplus and gained the weight back. This brings us back to your belief system. If you believe a program is "just for a short period of time," then you are setting yourself up for disappointment. If you work the program for the first twenty-one days and see great results, you will be motivated to continue and to adopt many of my recommendations as new habits that will keep the weight falling off.

crept up? I bet it does. The majority of Petites I have worked with say the same thing: "My weight just keeps slowly going up." Stick with me and believe in the power of The Math and you will quickly see the scale heading down.

Counting Calories

But, you say, I don't want to have to count calories; it's just too hard. This is an excuse that totally piggybacks on the previous paragraphs. I don't hear this from Petites who are successfully managing their weight. I hear it from Petites who are struggling with their weight. I have to be honest and tell you, it's really not that hard at all. You simply have to improve upon what I call your "caloric awareness."

You know the drill; you have to read labels. I bet there are truly only about thirty or forty food products that you buy all the time. I know that's about it for me, and I'm feeding myself and my two children half the time. If you read the label—once—you are done, and you have given yourself the tools to drop the weight.

There are two parts of the label that you should read:

1. Calories per serving.

2. Servings per container, which is just as important.

The servings per container are so important because many of you may be eating far more than one serving. The classic example is frozen yogurt or ice cream. There are four servings in the classic pint-size package, and that serving is generally one-half cup. Ladies, that's not a lot of yogurt or ice cream. You may be eating as many as two, three, or four servings and not even realizing that it equals 500 to 600 calories, or half your total calories for the day! Once you have a true understanding of your portions, your new belief system will translate to more successful behaviors.

This is only for the foods that you are purchasing and consuming at home. In chapter 6, I will give you all the tools you need to eat out successfully, enjoy yourself, and stay on plan.

Right now, I want you to fill out your own equation. If you don't want to get out your calculator, then please go to the Internet. It should take less than one minute for you to see your results. These numbers are going to make weight loss a whole lot easier, as you now have what I call "The Data."

Beating Bloat

You may be wondering how you are going to lose three to five pounds a week for the first twenty-one days if the math tells you that you are probably going to lose closer to two. That actually brings us back to the math again, as I am positive you are carrying pounds of water bloat. I said earlier that I didn't want you to lose water and muscle, but instead want you to lose only fat. That is true, but water "bloat" is a different story.

Where does water bloat come from? There are two culprits: sodium and excessive intake of processed carbohydrates. With regard to sodium (or salt), you may never even pick up a saltshaker. I bet the majority of you don't do that. But, unfortunately, there is sodium in so many foods that it's staggering. If, with any regularity, you are consuming fast food, processed foods, or fat-free carbohydrates, you are consuming a staggering amount of sodium. When they take the fat out of cookies, cakes, or muffins (which are really a form of cake), they pump them up with sodium to make them taste better. This is also true of many soups, unless they are the low-sodium version—and the list goes on. That sodium causes you to bloat, or appear puffy, since excessive salt intake causes you to retain water.

You know what I am talking about; you may feel it in your fingers (your rings are tight), in your shoes, and even see it around your eyes. You may be shocked to realize that, even as a Petite, you are carrying between three and seven pounds of water bloat, depending on your present body weight. You have been unknowingly carrying this extra weight in bloat for years. Water bloat is that much more prevalent in Petites, because the whiplash of sodium hits you harder than it does taller girls. With my eating and drinking plan in this book, you will immediately see that bloat disappear and, as long as you keep following my eating rules going forward, you will keep that water bloat off.

Processed carbohydrates also cause serious water bloat. When you consume too many processed carbohydrates—white bread, rice, potatoes, pasta, cookies, candy, sugar—your body holds more water, since certain carbs bind with water in the cells of your body. Think of a sponge filled with water. It's heavy. That's what happens when you are filled up with the wrong carbs. The minute you eliminate them, it's like wringing out a wet sponge. It becomes light and airy. That, too, will be you. By bringing the "wrong" carbs down and replacing them with the "right" ones, you will lose that water bloat. I will give you all these details in chapter 4. Just know that with your smaller stature, that "bloat" shows on you more than on other women. Bloat must be abolished!

That is why, in the first twenty-one days of my plan, you will really see the scales drop fast. And as I said, by continuing with these behaviors, you will keep the bloat off for good.

The second reason why the scales will go down quickly is because I am going to give you an intelligent internal "cleansing." Now, I want to be perfectly clear about this. I *strongly* dislike virtually every "cleansing" product sold. They place your body in "starvation" mode and that results in a diminished metabolism (and sheds your muscle, which is something you *never* want to do). That's exactly the same thing that happens when you skip meals, especially breakfast. After this ridiculous "cleansing" is over, you will instantly gain all your weight back and it will all be fat. You probably will gain even more weight, since your metabolism is now severely diminished. I've seen women, many of them Petites, lose ten pounds in two weeks, and then regain fifteen pounds in the next three weeks. Why? Because they destroyed their metabolisms.

Fabulous Fiber

For years, Petites have told me about issues with irregularity. I theorize that their smaller size makes this more of an issue. I wonder if that applies to you and, quite frankly, I bet it does. Most Petites don't even know what it feels like to be regular, which I describe as having at least one or two bowel movements each day.

My eating plan relies heavily on high-fiber foods in the form of fruits and vegetables, the right whole-wheat or whole-grain carbohydrates, and nuts. Fiber gives you the "natural" cleansing your body wants, not an artificial one that lasts just a few days. Fiber should be one of the cornerstones of your eating plan. That will get your body "moving" again in the right way.

That is also why I insist that you consume approximately three grams of fiber supplement about fifteen minutes before your dinner. You may mix the supplement with water or consume one of the tablet variety. It doesn't matter to me. All that matters is that you make consuming fiber a priority in the future. I include it for you in the twenty-one-day eating plan, but I strongly urge you to continue the same behavior in the future. Fiber helps keep you regular, lean, and full—full in the good way, as in "not hungry."

Fiber is a great tool for warding off hunger for two reasons. First, it helps fill your stomach. It's heavy and big. Then, the magic of fiber is that most of the calories pass through your body without being absorbed. That makes it a miracle food. The second reason I love fiber is that it regulates blood sugar and keeps it at an even level. You don't want your blood sugar to plummet or get too high. You want it to stay constant, and consuming adequate fiber enables that. The next chapter will really drive this issue home, but know for now that fiber plays a starring role in regulating blood sugar. Again, the issue of blood sugar is so important because it is directly linked to hunger, and I have established that hunger is Public Enemy #1 for Petites.

Need another big plus to consuming more fiber? By getting everything moving more efficiently, you will almost instantly flatten out your stomach and feel leaner. Your clothes, especially the waistbands, will feel looser. Yes! That's the direction we want to go. There can easily be four to five pounds of excess weight just hanging out in your intestines and digestive system. We are going to eliminate that, immediately. That's how the scale will head south so quickly. When you continue to follow the principles of my eating plan, that weight will never come back.

Think back to the baby pool. What happens when leaves start to fall into the pool? They plug up the filter and slow the whole cleaning process. If the same number of leaves drop into the bigger, Olympic-size pool, it may not be such a big deal. But you are that little pool. Anything negative is going to impact you to a greater extent.

Throughout the rest of the book, I am going to keep coming back to this math. The numbers add up, so be sure to use them to your advantage! Understanding this math is a huge step toward weight-loss success for every Petite.

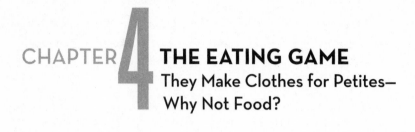

CHAPTER 4 **THE EATING GAME**
They Make Clothes for Petites—
Why Not Food?

Now that you understand The Math of Petite weight loss, you can use your newfound math skills to learn the most effective way to eat—a way that satisfies you both physically and mentally. You can learn to manage your hunger.

Hunger is a feeling you should avoid at all costs and hunger is especially detrimental to Petites.

- Hunger and overeating go hand in hand. Going back to our pool analogy, your baby pool is going to experience more damage from the overfilling, or overeating, when you let hunger take over.

- The *wrong* foods—the foods that cause hunger—are more detrimental to your body because you are smaller. Once you are chemically "fired up" and starving (generally because your blood sugar has plummeted from a lack of food), you will not only reach for too much food, generally you will reach for too much of the *wrong* foods. That will be even more detrimental to you as a Petite. Think of it as medication; doctors prescribe medication according to your size. As a Petite, you can't handle the same size dose that a taller person can. So a low-quality food is going to affect your hunger *and* your weight that much more.

The following eating rules represent the foundation of my eating plan for Petites that will keep satiety up and hunger down.

Protein

Protein is essential to this successful eating plan—more so than with any other weight-loss plan. I recommend that you consume approximately 35 percent of your total calories in protein. The upper limit to the majority of other weight-loss plans is 30 percent. I go that extra 5 percent as it will be protein comprised of the "good" fat, and not the artery-clogging saturated fat that should be kept to a minimum because of potential health issues. I have increased your percentage of protein because protein *is* the most difficult food to digest. This is actually good, as it will give you a more lasting feeling of satiety and thus ward off hunger. Here's how it works.

> ***Satiety is the key element to avoiding hunger.***
> *By keeping satiety mechanisms fired up through what and when you eat, you can minimize hunger, so that you eat for all the right reasons. Remember, eating breakfast is the first, most essential step to enhancing satiety and eradicating hunger.*

Think of protein as a woman's pearl necklace, with each individual pearl representing an amino acid. There are twenty individual amino acids or building blocks to protein. The body manufactures ten non-essential amino acids, while the remaining ten essential amino acids must be supplied by food. When you consume the necklace (a protein chain of essential amino acids), your stomach has to work hard to break the necklace apart. That "hard work" takes a good deal of time, and more time in your stomach translates into a more lasting feeling of satiety. That's very important for Petites, as some of you need to keep your total daily calories down in the 1100-calorie range on certain days.

In addition, protein has a very high thermic effect, which is defined as the incremental energy expenditure it takes to turn the food that you consume into fuel for energy (that's good) or storage (that's bad). Simply put, the thermic effect is the amount of calories it takes to bite, chew, and swallow food, plus the amount needed to process it—digest it, transport it, metabolize it, and store it. Protein has a thermic effect estimated as high as 30 percent. That means that 100 calories of protein actually requires as many as 30 calories for processing, leaving only 70 calories for your body to use. That's *good*! For the record, fat has a thermic effect of only 2 to 3 percent. That means that 100 fat calories consumed become 97 or 98 calories for your body to use or store. That's *bad*! In addition, protein helps maintain lean muscle tissue when restricting calories and losing body weight—and making sure that the weight lost is all fat! This is somewhat complicated, so let me break it down.

When you lose weight without my exercise program, you will lose approximately 60 to 70 percent fat and 30 to 40 percent muscle. Remember:

Lean Muscle Up = Metabolism Up

Research proves that the more protein you consume when restricting calories, or dieting, the more muscle you will spare. Therefore, you will keep your metabolism up while shedding pounds of fat. Since you know that muscle is the engine to a Petite's metabolism, you want to do everything in your power to minimize the loss of lean muscle tissue.

There has been a great deal of debate over the health benefits/costs of eggs and it appears that the benefits are clearly winning out. You will notice that there are a lot of eggs in the breakfasts in your eating plan. I have encouraged egg consumption for my Petites for years and truly believe they speed up weight loss by tipping "satiety" and avoiding hunger later in the day. A joint study at Saint Louis University and Wayne State University showed that eating eggs at breakfast resulted in 264 fewer calories being eaten each day and 418 fewer calories in a complete twenty-four-hour period.[1] If you eat 264 fewer calories a day for a year, you will lose twenty-seven and a half pounds—a year. That's a huge amount of weight loss.

This research was particularly interesting as the participants all ate the same calorie count for breakfast. The researchers theorize that the protein and fat in the eggs enabled this group to be less hungry—or as I would put it, the fat and protein helped to tip satiety levels. In addition, data from the Nurses' Health Study showed that the risk of increased cholesterol, heart disease, or stroke did not increase with egg consumption.

Now, let me be clear—this does not mean that eating protein will result in increasing your lean muscle tissue. That will only happen with my exercise program. But, when you restrict calories or diet, consuming adequate protein will result in *less* muscle loss with my exercise plan. I will all but guarantee that you will keep your muscle, but—just to be extra careful—I am going to increase your protein intake to be safe and smart.

Fat

The next fuel source I want to explore is *fat*. Of your total calories each day, you will receive approximately 25 percent of them from fat. Fat has gotten a *very* bad rap in the past two decades. Around the late 1980s, everyone said, "avoid fat—eat fat-free—eating fat will make you fat." The food companies then jumped on the "fat-free" bandwagon and churned out products that reduced the fat by stuffing products full of sugar and simple, refined carbohydrates to make up for the loss of fat. Later in this chapter, you will learn my thoughts on simple, refined carbs and sugars (it isn't good) and the fact that fat is good—if it's the right kind in the appropriate portion. You should also note that the fat-free belief system that came out of the late 1980s correlated with our obesity epidemic exploding—literally. That correlation comes as no surprise when you learn more about what simple, processed carbs and sugars do to our bodies and to our hunger.

There are two kinds of fat. The first, saturated fat, is what you need to minimize or avoid as much as possible, as this is the type of fat that increases the risk of heart disease as well as other illnesses. Saturated fats are found in fatty meats, butter, full-fat dairy products, egg yolks, the skin in animal protein (though there is a very, very small amount in boneless, skinless chicken and turkey,

> **Most people hear the words "better for you" and take that to mean "more is better."** Not true at all—and especially not true for you, Petites! If you are pouring olive oil all over your food (one tablespoon of olive oil is 120 calories and 100 percent fat) and pounding avocado (again, it's a good fat, but you only need a little) believing that you are making a healthy choice, you are sabotaging your desire to lose weight. I will help you to keep that from happening.

which is in your eating plan), and some processed and many fast foods. Not only is there fat in some of animal protein skin and fatty meat, there is also partially hydrogenated fat in some processed and fast foods that makes them even more lethal. Saturated fat should not constitute more than 10 percent of your daily caloric intake. In this eating plan, you will eat only 10 percent of your calories from saturated fat, as I totally agree with all the research. Saturated fat should be avoided—especially by Petites, since you are smaller and an average serving can cause more damage to you given your size.

Unsaturated fats, on the other hand, can lower cholesterol and aid in the reduction of heart disease. But don't be fooled, as these are still fats and that means they are high in calories. Unsaturated fats come from plants like peanuts, olives, corn, soybeans, and sunflowers. And, although they are *better* for you than saturated fats, remember my discussion about Addies, as they do fall into that category.

Simple Carbohydrates

Now, let's go on to how carbohydrates play into this eating plan. In the last decade, since the resurgence of the old Atkins diet, carbs have been vilified. That is so wrong, as most people are lumping all carbs into the same category. I want to introduce you to what I believe the three categories of carbohydrates should be.

The first category is processed, simple, refined, or "white" carbs. These carbs (they are generally white, which is why I added that name to the list) are pretty much the exact same thing, so don't get confused by the various names. Let's just call them the Evil Carbs. These evil carbohydrates have had all of the natural nutrients and fiber removed, which is why the name "simple" applies. They have been stripped of all their good, natural components, including fiber, which I have established as critically important to your success. They are what your mother may have referred to as "empty" calories, as they don't possess many vitamins or nutrients (if any). They are being blamed for a large part of our current obesity epidemic, as many people I know, especially Petites, consume them in very large quantities, unaware of their danger. Most people unfortunately rely on "evil" carbs because they are inexpensive, convenient (you can see and smell them everywhere), and easy to eat (how hard is it to open a bag of chips or a candy bar?). But they offer no nutritional value. The list of these carbs includes all white bread, bagels, pasta, rice, and chips, as well as sweet items like cookies, cake, and candy. And top off the list with the most evil of all "evil" carbs—liquid calories in the form of sports drinks, soda, and juice.

Why are these carbs so evil? Well, because the majority of these processed, simple, refined, or "white" carbs are what I refer to as a "quick empty" from the stomach.

All food turns to glucose in the bloodstream, which is then used for fuel (energy). For some, however, this may unfortunately be stored as body fat. It all depends on how you manipulate your "calories in minus calories out" equation. When you consume one of these evil carbohydrates, they very quickly empty into your bloodstream as glucose and spend very little time in your stomach. Again, that's why they are called "simple"—because all the good stuff has been stripped away, so your stomach has very little work to do. You want food to stay in your stomach (that's what protein does, since it is difficult to digest) and slowly empty into your bloodstream. But these evil carbs don't do that.

Insulin and the Blood-Sugar Dance

A "quick empty" is a major problem when it comes to hunger, which you are trying to avoid. A "quick empty" will lead to a big insulin surge. The human body is very efficient. It frequently operates in a "you do this and I'll do that" manner, generally to help it operate smoothly and in a balanced rhythm. That's good, and balance is truly what you want for your body. But that balance has to be used to your advantage and, in this instance, it's to your disadvantage. The "blood-sugar dance" is something that you want to manipulate *properly* and not let get extreme. You want your blood-sugar response to seem more like "easy listening" than "heavy metal rock." The goal of the blood-sugar dance is to maintain a slow, steady stream of food emptying from your stomach and turning into glucose for your body to use. That keeps hunger to a minimum, as your mind and body keep saying to each other: "Okay, there's a steady flow of glucose coming our way. No need to ask—*hunger*—for more."

Your ultimate partner in the blood-sugar dance is insulin. When blood sugar enters the bloodstream in a slow, "easy listening" way, the pancreas releases insulin in a similar way. Think of insulin as the drawbridge that allows the glucose to enter your cells for energy, or fuel. Most of this storage occurs in the liver and muscles. Without insulin to guide the way for glucose to enter, the sugar runs amok and causes tremendous damage to your body *and* to your desire to lose weight. I will elaborate on this in a moment.

Virtually all food turns to glucose, so that is not the issue. What is the issue is how quickly your food empties from your stomach and turns to glucose. Your goal is to consume foods that *slowly* leave the stomach and turn to glucose. When you consume a simple carb as a "stand-alone" food—which means you are not combining it with other fats or proteins, as when you get up first thing in the morning and grab breakfast—that's good. But if breakfast is a white bagel—that's bad. You get the unwanted "quick empty." A quick empty is *not* advantageous, as it will be interpreted by your body as a big "heavy metal" sugar party in your bloodstream. Your body doesn't want to be the host of that big sugar party and wants to shut it down quickly. That prompts your pancreas to push out a big insulin surge that pulls all that sugar out of your bloodstream.

Think of what happened when your parents came home early from vacation to find you throwing a big summer bash for 150 of your closest friends. They threw the lights on, killed the music (heavy metal?), and said "everyone out!" That's what your body does to the big sugar surge; it makes the pancreas secrete insulin to do its dirty work and get the sugar out fast. The human body is very, very smart. It knows that too much sugar in your bloodstream is a negative. Why is that so bad? *Hunger.*

Hunger and Energy

When you get that big insulin surge after your blood sugar is overly elevated, you *crash*, as the insulin strips all the sugar out of your bloodstream. I know you have probably felt this in the past. You just feel wiped out. What most people then do is reach for another processed carbohydrate. That's why those brownies you avoided all day suddenly become irresistible at 3:30, or you find yourself lured to the "break room"—a carb-lovers, "vending-machine fantasy." When you do this, you hit your body with another sugar surge, followed by another insulin surge and another crash. You spend far too much time each day on the sugar/insulin highway and that leads you to overeat—constantly. Since hunger is the enemy, when you regulate your blood sugar, you are well on your way to minimizing it—and your hunger and your weight. These carbs are the major culprits. They are also generally packed with calories, so not only do they induce hunger, they come with a great deal of caloric damage.

But carbs do more than promote hunger. Processed, refined, simple, or "white" carbs also annihilate energy levels. Why, you are thinking, would my energy level be important? Isn't this a weight-loss book? Yes, but you *need* energy. Remember our weight-loss equation—calories in minus calories out. First, to reduce calories in, you need the energy to make the right choices. Come on, you know what your decisions are like when you are exhausted. I don't have to dwell on that point. You reach for terrible things because you are too tired and think that a sugary fat-filled donut is going to give you the energy to power through. Second, to optimize calories out, you need the energy to work out *and* the energy to keep moving throughout the day. My most successful Petites move around a lot each day. They move for between sixty and ninety minutes a day. So do all the Petites following my program. This is also born out by the Seven Behaviors of Successful Weight Loss.

Now, that movement isn't exercise alone, nor should it be. Exercise should just be a small portion of your daily movement and it doesn't have to happen every day. But I know that Petites who have successfully followed my plan and lost weight possess more energy and *therefore* move more and burn more calories during their everyday lives. I'm not talking about a ten-mile hike. Just getting up to fill your tea or coffee mug or standing up at home when you are on the phone can make a difference. We have to manipulate that equation to your advantage.

You are the one telling your body to store fat. Excessive insulin in the bloodstream will make your body store more body fat. Insulin is basically a "storage" hormone. It shunts glucose into your cells, muscles, liver, etc. When you have too much insulin constantly circulating in your bloodstream (as a result of your repeated consumption of simple carbs), this promotes the accumulation of body fat. We know from the introduction that we are in the "fat-loss" business. Why, therefore, are we teaching—better yet, *demanding*—that your body store more and more fat by prompting a big insulin surge? This is not your goal as a Petite. *Your* regulation of *your* insulin will keep this from happening. That is why I want you to be so careful to avoid processed carbs whenever possible.

Inflammation

And what about your overall health? From my experience, good health and weight loss generally go hand in hand. In many instances, I find that health issues lead to weight gain, since you are in bed or unable to move around and are at the mercy of the easiest, most inexpensive foods—simple carbs. Americans across all geographic regions, socio-economic groups, and education levels are, well, "leveling" their health when it comes to rampant, internal inflammation. Simple carbs cause significant inflammation. According to Bharat B. Aggarwal, Ph.D. and Professor of Cancer Research and Cancer Medicine and Chief of the Cytokine Research Laboratory at the University of Texas M. D. Anderson Cancer Center, "Most chronic diseases have been found to be a result of too much inflammation, including cancer, heart attacks, diabetes, and Alzheimer's disease."[2]

Think of a sunburn or a burn you experienced when you grabbed a hot curling iron by mistake (my son, Evan, did that when he was four). What transpired? Well, the affected area became red and inflamed. That is what is going on in your body, internally, and for some people, all the time. You are "on fire," and not in the Dara Torres "swimming for the gold" positive sort of performance way. Your organs, cells, you name it, are virtually lit up, puffed up, swollen, and on fire because of what you are doing to them. This will lead to disease, illness, and accelerated aging, not to mention feeling terrible.

As a Petite, your body cannot withstand this tsunami of inflammation. You are smaller, therefore it is going to affect you more. Think of inflammation the way you think of alcohol. A few drinks may impact you far more than a larger person given your smaller size. You may have experienced that in the past. So the inflammatory response will hit you that much more as well. I have noticed for years that my smaller clients are getting hit with more autoimmune diseases like rheumatoid arthritis and celiac disease than my larger ones. I strongly believe that is because their bodies are more delicate and can't take the assault in the same way my larger clients can. This applies to inflammation as well.

A big—and I mean *big*—reason for this inflammation is simple, processed carbs. I know this is a weight-loss book, but you should be informed that these carbs I am asking you to shun are not only killing your desire to lose weight. They may be literally killing *you*.

And remember, as a Petite, these simple carbs will inflame you more than they will a taller person.

Complex Carbohydrates

The second category of carbohydrates is complex carbs—whole wheat and whole grain. While I said I truly want you to avoid the first category, the simple carbs, I'm not asking you to avoid whole-wheat and whole-grain carbohydrates, but I do want you to use them sparingly. Why?

First of all, these whole-wheat and whole-grain carbs are clearly better for your insulin response and the accompanying hunger. These carbs have more fiber and have not been stripped of other nutrients and vitamins. Therefore, they will stay in your stomach longer and slowly empty into your bloodstream as they become glucose. That's clearly better than the simple response.

Second, whole-wheat and whole-grain carbohydrates have been found to regulate hunger hormones effectively and tip satiety mechanisms. Two of the compounds in whole-wheat and whole-grain carbohydrates—fiber and resistant starch (which acts like fiber in the large intestine)—both appear to play a role in tipping this mechanism.[3]

I bet whole-grain and whole-wheat carbohydrates sound pretty great to you, but there is a big reason why Petites have to use them sparingly. Whole-wheat and whole-grain carbohydrates generally pack a lot of calories. I bet you thought that seven-grain bread was better than white bread. True? Yes and no. Yes, because it's better because it won't cause as rapid an insulin response. No, because it may pack many more calories than a simple carb. Since this is a weight-loss book, I have to help you manage hunger and drop your caloric intake.

Now, complex carbs do possess a higher thermic effect—some estimates place it as high as 20 percent. Therefore, 100 calories of whole wheat or whole grain, complex carbs, may only become 80 calories for use in the body. That clearly is a plus. But the minus is that, sometimes, the calorie counts of these products jump so rapidly that even a higher thermic effect cannot minimize the calorie damage. You will see in the actual eating plan that you rarely get more than a half-cup of brown rice or one piece of bread. By keeping your consumption of whole-grain and whole-wheat carbs on the lower side, you will lose weight faster, while still deriving many of the benefits of these carbs. For Petites, a little goes a long way.

How do you minimize these whole-wheat and whole-grain carbs? You read labels. It will take you less than ten seconds to check out the label on a loaf of whole-grain or whole-wheat bread or a package of brown or wild rice. With regard to pasta, I have to be honest. For your first twenty-one days, I want you to eliminate it. It is simply so densely caloric that a few strands add up to hundreds of calories very quickly. In the future, you can have some, but you'll have to be mindful of the portion.

Fruits and Vegetables

The third category of carbohydrates is fruits and vegetables. *Love* them both. As you will soon see, they are the foundation of my weight-loss and eating plan. But I want to take a moment to clear up some confusion with regard to fruit, as it has recently been given a bad, undeserved rap.

Quick. Who do you know who is overweight as the result of excessive tomato consumption? Did your BFF call you last night to say: "Oh, I'm out of control! Help me. I gorged on fresh peaches from the Farmer's Market all night. I worry I may do it again today." Or better yet, when was the last time you were at a restaurant or party and witnessed someone gorging on apples or pears? Does this possibly sound as crazy to you as it does to me? Everyone keeps saying to me: "Jim, what is your take on fruit? Should we be avoiding it? I hear it is terribly high in sugar." My answer—*no*. The truth is that some fruits have a higher glycemic index than others. The glycemic index is a measure of how quickly a food turns to sugar, which we know is really fast for simple carbs. To give you an example, pretzels, a classic simple carb, have a glycemic index of 83. An apple's index is 38. While there are some fruits—watermelon, pineapple, plums—that do inch up higher, they are still wonder foods because they are packed with fiber, water, vitamins, and nutrients.

I eat fruit all the time and urge lean Petites to eat it all the time as well. Just make it a point to combine fruit with protein, which is what I have set out for you in the plan. When you combine protein with your fruit, the glycemic index plummets because protein stays so long in the stomach. A classic example is a piece of apple and a tablespoon of peanut butter. That will make all the food that is in your stomach—both the fruit and the protein—turn to glucose more slowly, stabilizing the blood-sugar response. And we already know that we want food to take a long time in the stomach, as that will keep you feeling full longer and ward off hunger.

Please don't believe the hype that fruit is a "no-no." It's "not not."

Now, since I have addressed the fruit issue, I can lump fruits and vegetables together. Unfortunately, the Centers for Disease Control and Prevention developed a National Action Plan in 2005 to increase public health through increased consumption of fruits and vegetables. That makes sense, as they are packed with vitamins and nutrients that improve health *and* facilitate weight loss. Unfortunately, the report was *not* good. The goal was to get Americans to consume two cups of fruit and two and a half cups of vegetables each day. That doesn't sound like that much to me. If you can believe it, however, only 6 percent of Americans hit this goal, which I happen to think is very, very low. Think about that. Only 6 percent of all Americans eat two cups of fruit and two and a half cups of vegetables a day. Are you hitting this goal? Only 6 percent of you are.

I consider fruits and vegetables a Petite's best friend for three reasons.

The first is *fiber*. Fiber is one of the essential components that slows the emptying of all foods from your stomach. That slow emptying will minimize the insulin response (and create that "easy listening" environment). That keeps ramped-up insulin levels from making you hungry and causing you to store fat. I like that a lot and so should you. Unfortunately, the average American only eats half of the twenty-eight to thirty-eight grams of fiber recommended. In my plan, you are going to get to that level each day, whether with food or with the help of a fiber supplement.

I strongly urge you all to eat three grams of fiber, either in a powder that you mix with water or in a tablet, approximately fifteen minutes before your dinner. Not only is the fiber great for many reasons, but your dinner is going to be your *smallest* meal of the day, which will be a change for many of you. That fiber consumption prior to the meal will enable you to feel full on less food, which is the whole goal of this eating plan. Trust me, it works. In addition, the power of the "slow empty" will keep you feeling full.

The second reason that fiber is your best friend is that it is heavy. There are a number of research studies that prove that the heavier the food—like fruits and vegetables—the more you feel full. I believe that to be true and have seen it firsthand when I instruct a Petite to eat more fruits and vegetables. She comes back lower in weight *and* claiming that she is regularly feeling full.

Think about that for a moment. Pretzels and chips are the perfect example. Most struggling Petites have confessed to me that they were eating a lot of simple carbs like pretzels and chips (both quickly turn to sugar) and that they never felt full. They just kept eating and eating. Then they replaced those simple, lightweight carbs with the right carbs like fruits and vegetables and dropped weight—fast. That's exactly what you are going to do.

The third reason is regularity. We know that fiber helps keep everything moving and regularity will lead to a flat belly. Especially as a Petite, I want to lean you out in the midsection. We are going for that tight, hourglass figure, and that requires a leaned-out midsection. Regularity will lead to a more efficient metabolism (got to *love* that). You've no doubt heard the expression "a well-oiled machine." Well, we want you optimally taking in food and eliminating it efficiently and regularly. I have said to hundreds of successful Petites: "So, tell me, are we *moving* more these days?" They look at me and say: "How did you know? I haven't gone this much in years. I wondered if there was something wrong with me." No; not at all. You *want* this regularity for weight loss.

Regularity also will eliminate toxins from your body more effectively. I know, I know, this is a weight-loss book, but in a less toxic environment, you will feel better, have more energy, *and* immediately appear to lean out. In chapter 7, we are going to delve into the issue of water balance. For now, trust me that the more I can lean you out and get rid of the water bloat, the better you will look and feel. That alone will keep you coming back to this plan for more information and success.

Just so we are clear on the issue of carbs, I want you to:

- Avoid simple carbs.

- Cut way back on whole-wheat and whole-grain carbs.

- Push the vegetables and fruit and don't be afraid of fruit!

Snacking

Since you now have a better understanding of the role of protein, fat, and carbs, I now want to address the issue of snacking. I'm a big fan of snacking, especially for you. Let's look at why.

We just talked about blood sugar and energy with regard to the insulin response to certain foods. You don't want to consume foods like simple carbs that lead to excessive glucose in your bloodstream. That is followed by a big insulin surge, which causes your blood sugar to plummet, making you totally devoid of energy and ravenously looking for something else to eat. You may feel fatigue, nausea, and dizziness and just want to put your head down and crash. To avoid this, smart snacking comes into play. By snacking and not letting your blood-sugar levels get too low, you enable insulin to do its job most effectively and you keep your energy levels up for making better food choices, and for activity and exercise.

Blood sugar also affects hunger. Energy levels plummet with low blood sugar, and low blood sugar leads to hunger. And you now know that hunger is Public Enemy #1 for Petites. My goal is for you to feel hungry *only* first thing in the morning, after you have been on an eight or more hour fast. That's the time to feel hungry and why breakfast is so important. But, for the rest of the day, you should never feel hunger, and smart snacking keeps that from happening.

Now, to be clear, there is research that snacking is a major contributor to our obesity epidemic. I can understand this line of reasoning if you are snacking on abundant, "quick empty" processed carbs in the form of cookies, cake, or candy, which I refer to as *sugar crap cubed*. Add to that chips, pretzels, cheese curls, pork rings, fried crap, and salted whatever and you are talking about major calories doing all the wrong things to your caloric intake, energy levels, hunger, and health. That's not the snacking I'm talking about.

Calorie Cycling

This is where calorie cycling comes in. I have always been deeply committed to research and my own experience, and to my clients' weight loss. The subject of calorie cycling is almost exclusively based on my experience working directly with clients and, most important, my work with Petites.

I started exploring calorie cycling many years ago when I witnessed both men and women, Petites and Non-Petites, in astonishing shape. I mean, the women in particular looked like the cover of *Sports Illustrated's* swimsuit edition. For the record, I like the fact that this magazine puts athletic-looking, lean women on the cover and not unattractive, insanely skinny supermodels. I asked these women what their secret was, and time after time I heard about some type of calorie cycling. It was explained by some as "high days" and "low days." I test everything on myself, so I gave it a try. I found it very effective for me, as a six-foot-tall, 175-pound man. I played with the balance of high and low days and found that one low day, followed by one high, worked best for me.

Then I started bringing the concept to my clients in Chicago and New York. Again, I saw weight *and* fat shedding off my female clients. I remember one Petite who seemed very down during one of our workouts. She said: "Jim, I've lost twenty pounds, but you and I agree that I have another twenty to go. I feel as if it's now coming off very slowly and it's hard for me to stay motivated and not want to cheat. What can we do?" Immediately I said: "We are going to do a major overhaul of your eating plan and get you to a calorie cycle." She first looked at me oddly, and then I explained the concept. Just the thought of getting to eat more on certain days was appealing. I decided that, given her smaller size, she should have two low days followed by one high day, because of the math of weight loss. Within the first eight days, she knocked off a solid four pounds. That's a lot of weight for a Petite in that short amount of time, but she said that her "low days" were now much easier. She said she had no desire to cheat, as she knew the high day was coming up shortly.

She lost all twenty pounds in a little over six weeks. We were both amazed by the ease and the outcome. Since then, I have always put Petite clients on the calorie cycle from the start.

The ratio I want you to follow is the same one I used for this Petite client: two low-calorie days (approximately 1100 calories a day) followed by one high-calorie day (approximately 1600 calories). The approximate ratio of protein (35 percent), carbohydrates (40 percent), and fat (25 percent) will remain the same. It's the total calories that will go up and down.

Cycling is critically important to you because:

1. It physically enables you to keep the calories down. You must bring your total calories consumed down lower than larger people. Remember our math. It's creating a caloric deficit that gets the weight off *and* the fat off. After two days of low-calorie eating, I want to reward you for the great work by giving you 500 more calories. Five hundred more calories is a lot of additional food.

2. It enables you to trick your metabolism. I established how important metabolism is to your weight-loss success. By cycling in a higher-calorie day every third day, you trick your metabolism into staying elevated. I have never had a problem with a Petite's metabolism slowing on this plan. And, I build in an advantage by coupling the right exercise program with this calorie cycling.

3. It mentally rewards you for keeping the calories down. While this may sound like a repeat of point 1, it's not. That dealt with the physical feeling. This deals with the psychological feeling. If you know that you are going to get a higher-calorie day, you say to yourself: "I can do this because I get a reward in a day or two." That fact, plus the fact that the scale is going down, will keep you right on this plan.

4. It makes eating out easier. While I will give you very specific details on eating out, clearly you will get more calories on your high-calorie day. Therefore, you can plan in your schedule when you are going to eat out according to what day you are on in this cycle. It's a great way to eliminate the deprived feeling that most people experience when on a weight-loss plan. And, it is a plan you can easily follow for continued success.

Now, let's translate this chapter's information into your actual eating plan for the next twenty-one days.

CHAPTER 5 THE EATING PLAN

Throughout this chapter, I outline in detail your twenty-one-day eating plan. This specialized plan is formulated for Petites and is very specific. Let's take a look at some of the components. While following this plan you are going to:

1. **Front-load calories.** You are going to eat your biggest meal of the day at breakfast. You will be leaving behind your flawed belief that you have to "save" your calories to use throughout the day. Eating your biggest meal at the beginning of your day is crucial for Petites. It just works. By giving it a try, you have nothing to lose—nothing but weight.

2. **Follow a very specific eating "allocation"** so that you stay mentally and physically full and ward off all hunger. You will be following a three-day cycle that includes two days of 1100 calories, followed by one day of 1600 calories.

   Your 1100-calorie-day meal allocation breaks down to:

   - 400 calories for breakfast
   - 300 calories for lunch
   - 300 calories for dinner

- 100 calories for a snack, which should always be in the mid to late afternoon around 3:00 or 4:00, depending on when you had lunch.

On the third day of each three-day cycle, your 1600-calorie day, I allow you a bigger dinner, since I think of this day as your "carrot" day to keep you on plan for the other two days. But, I also kept your breakfast high so that you continue to tip satiety mechanisms. On this day, you are going to enjoy:

- 500 calories for breakfast

- 400 calories for lunch

- 500 calories for dinner

- Two 100-calorie snacks

You may notice that you are only getting one snack on your 1100-calorie days. I like snacking, but on your 1100-calorie days, I only want you to snack once a day, in the mid to late afternoon. On the days that you receive two snacks, I generally would like to see one in the midafternoon and the second immediately after you exercise. I will even allow you to add one 100-calorie snack to your dinner, if that is something that appeals to you. You can do this twice during the first twenty-one days. There are certain things I feel you need to be rigid about and certain areas where you can relax.

But just to be clear, I don't want you flipping this eating plan and "back-loading" your calories at night. I feel that the research and my personal experience with "front-loading" are compelling enough to insist that you follow my advice. Plus, I give you a bigger dinner every three days. Isn't successful weight loss worth it? And you will be amazed, because you won't be hungry.

On this plan, you will consume more protein. In the past, I have generally recommended:

- 40 percent of your calories from carbohydrates

- 30 percent of your calories from protein

- 30 percent of your calories from fat

But in this plan, you are going to increase protein slightly at the expense of fat and eat approximately:

- 40 percent of your calories from carbohydrates

- 35 percent of your calories from protein

- 25 percent of your calories from fat

I said "approximately," as it is very difficult to hit these numbers perfectly each day. Just know that I am very close. I am going with these percentages for four reasons:

- The metabolic boost that comes from consuming more protein.

- The thermic effect of the protein, which translates to lower calories available for your body to use.

- The feeling of fullness that comes from consuming more protein.

- I want to get the fat percentage closer to what I have recommended for my most successful Petites—a level that is also reinforced by the research in the Seven Behaviors of Successful Weight Loss, which was 23 percent. The fat that you will be consuming will generally be in the food you are eating and does not fall into the Addie category, unless it is in very clear portion sizes.

Grocery List

Week 1

1 package Louis Rich Turkey Bacon

2 cups cut pineapple

1 package cheddar or colby cheese slices, low fat

12 eggs

2 sweet potatoes

sour cream, reduced fat

1 can pinto beans

3 heads fresh broccoli

2 sweet onions

1 large bag fresh spinach

low-fat French salad dressing

1 fresh lemon

1 oz feta cheese

1 4-oz filet of halibut

1 Oikos Organic Greek Yogurt, vanilla, 6 oz

1 container 2% cottage cheese

6 tomatoes

1 loaf Ezekiel 4:9 Sprouted Grain Bread

2 heads Romaine lettuce

Grey Poupon de Dijon mustard

1 bag brown rice

1 firm tofu, prepared with calcium sulfate and magnesium chloride (nigari)

scallops, raw, 3 units (2 large or 5 small)

2 cucumbers

1 bunch cilantro

1 fresh lime

1 mango

1 bunch asparagus

gallon 1% milk

1 small container oats

1 jar almond butter

1 fresh apple

1 small box raisins

cinnamon

small bag flaxseed

3 peppers—sweet, red, or green—fresh

Mrs. Dash Lemon Pepper Seasoning Blend

3 chicken breasts, no skin

1 bunch basil

1 package La Tortilla Factory Whole-Wheat Low-Carb Tortillas

2 6-oz filets of Atlantic salmon

1 small bottle teriyaki sauce

Mrs. Dash Garlic & Herb
Seasoning Blend

1 small box couscous

1 bag raw almonds

1 jar salsa

1 bunch scallions

1 can black beans

1 whole-wheat pita

1 lb deli turkey

1 oz Swiss cheese

1 bay leaf

1 bag carrots

1 bag celery

1 fresh garlic bulb

1 can northern beans

1 can Campbell's low-sodium
chicken broth

2 pints blueberries

2 cartons strawberries

1 bag walnuts

3 Fage 0% yogurt

1 lb On Gold Standard 100%
Whey Protein

3 tbs Parmesan cheese

1 bunch parsley

4 oz ground turkey

1 cantaloupe

1 small bottle balsamic vinegar

1 5-oz flank steak

1 kiwi

1 small container hummus

sweet corn, fresh

1 jalapeño

Week 2

1 banana

1 cup cherry tomatoes

1 4-oz filet of yellow fin tuna

1 cup snap peas

1 small bottle olive oil

1 bag carrots

3 heads Romaine lettuce

2 containers mushrooms

5 green/red peppers

7 chicken breasts, 34 oz total

1 can Campbell's low-sodium
chicken broth

1 bottle white wine

2 pints raspberries

1 pint blueberries

1 bag arugula

3 sweet onions

6 tomatoes

1 avocado

3 cucumbers

1 bunch radishes

1 small bag dried cranberries

12 eggs

1 large tub cottage cheese, 2% milk fat (not packed)

1 bag spinach

pine nuts

2 bunches asparagus

1 small jar sesame seeds

1 3-oz filet of Atlantic salmon

1 bag wheat bran muffins with raisins

1 kiwi

1 bag shrimp

1 can garbanzo beans

Sriracha chili sauce

fresh ginger root

8 slices deli turkey

1 can black beans

1 bag brown rice

gallon 1% milk

1 box Fiber One cereal

2 pints strawberries

3 tbsp tzatziki dip

alfalfa sprouts

1 bunch fresh dill weed

1 medium summer squash

1 5-oz filet of Atlantic salmon

1 lemon

1 medium zucchini

2 Laughing Cow Original Cheese

3 medium apples

1 hot chili pepper

chili powder

garlic powder

1 bunch of scallions

Week 3

3 jalapeños

1 bag shrimp

1 loaf Ezekiel 4:9 Sprouted Grain Bread

low-fat Philadelphia Herb & Garlic Cream Cheese

3 heads broccoli

1 6-oz filet of mahimahi, individually wrapped

1 4-oz filet of mahimahi, individually wrapped

5 Fage 0% yogurt

1 small jar Kraft fat-free mayo

1 can Tuna, Starkist Chunk White Albacore in Water

1 bag celery

1 4-oz pork tenderloin

4 fresh beets

1 pint raspberries

1 onion

2 pints strawberries

1 large green/red pepper

4 oz ground turkey

basil

Parmesan cheese, grated

10 brussels sprouts, cooked

1 dozen eggs

2% cottage cheese

1 can chickpeas

1 bag spinach

5 tomatoes

1 cucumber

2 oz goat cheese

1 lime

1 container mushrooms

soy sauce made from soy and wheat (shoyu), low sodium

1 block tofu, firm

bean sprouts

1 medium apple

2 pints blueberries

1 4-oz filet of yellow fin tuna

1 cup cherry tomatoes

snap peas

3 heads Romaine lettuce

1 eggplant

1 3-oz Atlantic salmon filet

1 banana

1 bag spinach

2 chicken breasts

4 oz beef skirt steak, lean

1 oz feta cheese

1 can water chestnuts

1 5-oz flank steak

Jim Karas Meal Plan 1100-1100-1600

Day 1

Breakfast: Turkey Bacon Scramble

	Protein	Fat	Carbs	Calories	Fiber, total dietary
Louis Rich Turkey Bacon (1 slice), 2 servings	4	5	0	70	0
Pineapple, fresh, 1 cup, diced	1	1	19	76	2
Cheddar or colby cheese, low fat, 2 slices (1 oz each)	14	4	1	98	0
Egg white, 2 servings	10	0	0	34	0
Karas Egg*, 1 serving	6	7	1	90	0
Meal Totals	**35**	**17**	**21**	**368**	**2**

Directions:

1. Coat the inside of a nonstick skillet with cooking spray.
2. Mix the egg whites and one egg together.
3. Scramble until fully cooked and top with turkey bacon, pineapple, and cheese.

---

* A Karas Egg is just a plain egg, a staple in this diet.

Lunch: Loaded Sweet Potato

	Protein	Fat	Carbs	Calories	Fiber, total dietary
Sweet potato, cooked, baked in skin, without salt, ½ medium (2" dia., 5" long, raw)	1	0	12	51	2
Sour cream, reduced fat, 2 tbsp	1	4	1	41	0
Beans, pinto, ⅗ cup	8	1	26	141	9
Cheddar or colby cheese, low fat, 1 slice (1 oz)	7	2	1	49	0
Broccoli, fresh, 3 spears (about 5" long)	3	0	5	26	3
Meal Totals	**20**	**7**	**45**	**308**	**14**

Directions:

1. Pierce the potato with fork and place in microwave for 5 minutes or until done.
2. Top the potato with pinto beans, sour cream, cheese, and broccoli spears.

Dinner: Grilled Halibut with Fresh Spinach Salad

	Protein	Fat	Carbs	Calories	Fiber, total dietary
Onions, raw, 5 rings	0	0	3	11	1
Spinach, fresh, 1 ½ cups	1	0	2	10	1
French salad dressing, low fat, 2 tbsp	0	2	7	44	0
Lemon, ½ fruit without seeds	1	0	6	11	3
Feta cheese, 1 oz	4	6	1	75	0
Halibut filet, 4 oz	30	3	0	159	0
Meal Totals	**36**	**11**	**19**	**310**	**5**

Directions:

1. Grill halibut filet until done and drizzle with lemon juice.
2. Combine spinach, onions, and feta, and drizzle with salad dressing.

Snack: Greek Yogurt

Oikos Organic Greek Yogurt, vanilla, 6 oz	15	0	12	110	0
Meal Totals	**15**	**0**	**12**	**110**	**0**
Daily Totals	**106**	**35**	**97**	**1096**	**19**

Day 2

Breakfast: Open-Face Breakfast BLT

	Protein	Fat	Carbs	Calories	Fiber, total dietary
Cottage cheese, 2% milk fat, 1 cup (not packed)	28	2	6	163	0
Tomato, red, ripe, raw, 1 medium whole (2 3/5" dia.)	1	0	6	26	1
Ezekiel 4:9 Sprouted Grain Bread (1 slice), 1 serving	4	1	15	80	3
Louis Rich Turkey Bacon (1 slice), 3 servings	6	7	0	105	0
Romaine lettuce (salad), 2 inner leaves	0	0	0	3	0
Grey Poupon de Dijon mustard, 1 tsp	0	0	0	5	0
Meal Totals	**39**	**10**	**27**	**382**	**4**

Directions:
1. Toast bread and top with mustard, bacon, lettuce, and tomato.
2. Have cottage cheese on the side.

Lunch: Cheesy Tofu Rice Bowl

	Protein	Fat	Carbs	Calories	Fiber, total dietary
Broccoli, fresh, 2 spears (about 5" long)	2	0	3	17	2
Brown rice, medium grain, 1/3 cup	1	1	15	72	1
Tofu, firm, prepared with calcium sulfate and magnesium chloride (nigari), half brick	13	7	5	125	1
Cheddar or colby cheese, low fat, 2 oz	14	4	1	98	0
Meal Totals	**30**	**12**	**24**	**312**	**4**

Directions:

1. Cook brown rice until done.
2. Steam broccoli and place in bowl with rice.
3. Take half brick of tofu and slice into small squares and add to bowl and top it with cheese.

Dinner: Seared Scallops with Mango Salsa

	Protein	Fat	Carbs	Calories	Fiber, total dietary
Scallops, raw, 3 units, 2 large or 5 small	15	1	2	79	0
Cucumber (peeled), 1 cup, pared, chopped	1	0	3	16	1
Cilantro, raw, 4 tbsp	0	0	0	0	0
Onions, raw, ½ cup, chopped	1	0	7	30	1
Lime juice, 1 lime yield	0	0	3	10	0
Mangoes, 1 cup, sliced	1	0	28	107	3
Asparagus, fresh, 15 spears, medium (5 ¼" to 7" long)	5	0	11	55	5
Meal Totals	**23**	**1**	**54**	**297**	**10**

Directions for Scallops:

1. Coat the inside of a nonstick pan with spray, turn to medium-high heat.
2. Sear scallops on each side for 3–4 minutes or until they have a golden crust.
3. Steam asparagus and serve with scallops.

Directions for the Salsa:

1. Cut the mangoes in small squares, along with the onions and cucumbers.
2. Place those items in a bowl and drizzle with lime juice and top with chopped cilantro.
3. Top the scallops with the fresh salsa.

Snack: Milk

Milk, 1%, 1 cup	8	2	12	110	0
Meal Totals	**8**	**2**	**12**	**110**	**0**
Daily Totals	**100**	**25**	**117**	**1101**	**18**

Day 3

Breakfast: Oatmeal with Apples, Raisins, and Almond Butter

	Protein	Fat	Carbs	Calories	Fiber, total dietary
Oats, ½ cup	5	2	52	150	8
Almond butter, 1 ¼ tbsp	3	12	4	127	1
Apple, fresh, ½ cup, quartered or chopped	0	0	10	37	2
Raisins, 1 small box (½ oz)	0	0	11	42	1
Cinnamon, ground, 1 tsp	0	0	2	6	1
Flaxseed, 2 tbsp	5	8	8	118	7
Meal Totals	**13**	**22**	**87**	**480**	**20**

Directions:

1. Cook oats until done.
2. Stir in almond butter and flaxseeds.
3. Top with apple and raisins and sprinkle cinnamon on top.

Lunch: Basil Chicken Wrap

	Protein	Fat	Carbs	Calories	Fiber, total dietary
Peppers, sweet, red, fresh, 1 cup, chopped	1	O	10	40	3
Mrs. Dash Lemon Pepper Seasoning Blend, ¼ tsp	O	O	O	O	O
Chicken breast, bone and skin removed, 6 oz	54	3	O	260	O
Onions, raw, 10 slices, thin	1	O	8	34	2
Basil, 3 leaves	O	O	O	O	O
La Tortilla Factory Whole Wheat Low-Carb Tortilla, 1 serving	5	2	10	50	7
Meal Totals	**61**	**5**	**28**	**384**	**12**

Directions:

1. Cook chicken breast until done, season with lemon pepper.
2. Slice chicken breast and place it in the wrap.
3. Add sliced peppers, onions, and three basil leaves.

Dinner: Teriyaki Salmon with Broccoli

	Protein	Fat	Carbs	Calories	Fiber, total dietary
Atlantic salmon filet, 6 oz	43	14	0	309	0
Broccoli, fresh, 6 spears (about 5" long)	6	1	10	52	6
Teriyaki sauce, 1 tbsp	1	0	3	16	0
Pineapple, fresh, 1 slice, thin (3 ½" dia. x ½" thick)	0	0	7	27	1
Mrs. Dash Garlic & Herb Seasoning Blend, ¼ tsp	0	0	0	0	0
Couscous, ½ cup, cooked	3	0	18	88	1
Meal Totals	**53**	**15**	**38**	**492**	**8**

Directions:

1. Coat the inside of a nonstick pan with spray; turn it on to medium heat.
2. Cook until fish easily flakes with a fork.
3. Top with teriyaki sauce and pineapple.
4. Steam broccoli and season it with garlic-and-herb seasoning blend.
5. Cook the couscous until done and place salmon on top of it.

Snack 1: Almonds
Snack 2: Milk

Almonds, 15	4	9	4	104	2
Milk, 1%, 1 cup	8	2	12	110	0
Meal Totals	**12**	**11**	**16**	**214**	**2**
Daily Totals	**139**	**53**	**169**	**1570**	**42**

Day 4

Breakfast: Breakfast Burrito

	Protein	Fat	Carbs	Calories	Fiber, total dietary
Cheddar or colby cheese, low fat, 1 oz	7	2	1	49	0
Salsa, ¼ cup	1	0	4	18	1
Scallions, raw, 1 tbsp chopped	0	0	0	2	0
Cilantro, raw, 1 tbsp	0	0	0	0	0
Whole-wheat tortilla, 1 serving	4	3	24	130	4
Egg white, 4 servings	20	0	1	68	0
Beans, black, ½ cup	8	0	20	114	7
Meal Totals	**40**	**5**	**50**	**381**	**12**

Directions:

1. Coat the inside of a nonstick pan with cooking spray.
2. Mix the egg whites, scallions, and black beans in a bowl and add to the pan.
3. Scramble until fully cooked.
4. Add the scramble to the tortilla and top with salsa, cilantro, and cheese.

Lunch: Swiss and Spinach Turkey Pita

	Protein	Fat	Carbs	Calories	Fiber, total dietary
Bread, pita, whole-wheat, ½ pita, large (6 ½" dia.)	3	1	18	85	2
Spinach, fresh, 2 cups	2	O	2	14	1
Turkey breast meat, 3 oz	15	1	4	88	O
Swiss cheese, 1 oz	8	8	1	107	O
Meal Totals	**28**	**10**	**25**	**294**	**3**

Directions:

1. Take half of a large whole-wheat pita and stuff with spinach, turkey breast meat, and Swiss cheese.
2. For some extra spice, squeeze some Sriracha hot chili sauce on top.

Dinner: Hearty Chicken and Bean Stew

	Protein	Fat	Carbs	Calories	Fiber, total dietary
Chicken breast, 4 oz	27	1	0	130	0
Spinach, fresh, 1 cup	1	0	1	7	1
Carrots, raw, ¼ cup, chopped	0	0	3	13	1
Celery, raw, 1 cup, diced	1	0	4	19	2
Garlic, 3 cloves	1	0	3	13	0
Beans, great northern, ½ cup	7	0	19	104	6
Campbell's low-sodium chicken broth, 1 cup	3	0	1	13	0
Meal Totals	**40**	**1**	**31**	**299**	**10**

Directions:

1. Cook chicken breast until done.
2. Slice chicken and place into medium saucepan with chicken broth.
3. Add one bay leaf.
4. Thinly slice the celery, carrots, and garlic and add to the pot.
5. Add the beans and spinach.
6. Let this simmer for 10 minutes or until all vegetables are cooked through.

Snack: Celery and Almond Butter

Almond butter, 1 tbsp	2	9	3	101	1
Celery, raw, 1 stalk, medium (7 ½"-8" long)	0	0	1	6	1
Meal Totals	**2**	**9**	**4**	**107**	**2**
Daily Totals	**110**	**25**	**110**	**1081**	**27**

Day 5

Breakfast: Fruit and Greek Yogurt

	Protein	Fat	Carbs	Calories	Fiber, total dietary
Blueberries, fresh, 1 cup	1	0	21	81	4
Strawberries, fresh, 10 medium (1 ¼" dia.)	1	0	8	36	3
Walnuts, ½ oz (14 halves)	2	9	2	95	1
Fage – 0%, 8 oz	20	0	9	120	0
On Gold Standard 100% Whey Protein, ½ serving	12	1	2	60	0
Meal Totals	**36**	**10**	**42**	**392**	**8**

Directions:

1. Put the Greek yogurt into a bowl.
2. Stir in half scoop of protein powder.
3. Top the yogurt with blueberries, strawberries, and walnuts.

Lunch: Mexican Loaded Sweet Potato

	Protein	Fat	Carbs	Calories	Fiber, total dietary
Sweet potato, cooked, baked in skin, without salt, 1 medium (2" dia., 5" long, raw)	2	0	24	103	4
Onions, raw, ¼ cup, chopped	0	0	3	15	1
Salsa, ⅛ cup	0	0	2	9	1
Sour cream, reduced-fat, 2 tbsp	1	4	1	41	0
Beans, black, ⅗ cup	9	1	24	136	9
Meal Totals	**12**	**5**	**54**	**304**	**15**

Directions:

1. Pierce the potato with fork and place in microwave for 5 minutes or until done.
2. Top the potato with black beans, sour cream, onions, and salsa.

Dinner: Turkey Meatballs with Homemade Tomato Sauce

	Protein	Fat	Carbs	Calories	Fiber, total dietary
Parmesan cheese, grated, 3 tbsp	6	5	1	68	0
Parsley, 10 sprigs	0	0	1	4	0
Garlic, 3 cloves	1	0	3	13	0
Red, ripe tomatoes, 2 medium whole (2 3/5" dia.)	3	1	12	59	4
Ground turkey, 93% lean, 4 oz	22	8	0	160	0
Meal Totals	**32**	**14**	**17**	**304**	**4**

Directions for Tomato Sauce:

1. Score the top of the tomatoes (cut 1-inch X on top).
2. Add tomatoes to a pot of boiling water.
3. Boil the tomatoes for 30 seconds to one minute, then place in a bowl of ice water to stop the cooking process.
4. Peel the tomatoes and finely chop them.
5. Spray a nonstick pan with cooking spray and add 2 cloves of finely chopped garlic on medium heat.
6. Sauté garlic until golden brown.
7. Add tomatoes to pan and gently mash them into a chunky sauce.

Directions for Meatballs:

1. In a bowl combine ground turkey, 1 clove of finely chopped garlic, chopped parsley, and 2 tbsp of Parmesan cheese.
2. Stir together contents of the bowl and roll the mixture into small meatballs.
3. Spray a nonstick pan with cooking spray and turn it on to medium heat.
4. Add meatballs.
5. Turn and rotate the meatballs until they are fully cooked.
6. Top the meatballs with sauce and sprinkle with 1 tbsp of Parmesan cheese.

Snack: Hard-Boiled Egg

	Protein	Fat	Carbs	Calories	Fiber, total dietary
Hard-boiled egg, 1 large	6	5	1	70	0
Meal Totals	**6**	**5**	**1**	**70**	**0**
Daily Totals	86	34	114	1070	26

Day 6

Breakfast: Fresh Fruit Protein Shake and Toast

	Protein	Fat	Carbs	Calories	Fiber, total dietary
Cantaloupe, ½ melon, medium (about 5" dia.)	2	1	23	97	2
Strawberries, fresh, 20 medium (1 ¼" dia.)	1	1	17	72	6
On Gold Standard 100% Whey Protein, 1 serving	24	1	3	120	0
Ezekiel 4:9 Sprouted Grain Bread (1 slice), 1 serving	4	1	15	80	3
Almond butter, 1 tbsp	2	9	3	101	1
Meal Totals	**33**	**13**	**61**	**470**	**12**

Directions:

1. Place cantaloupe, strawberries, and protein powder in a blender.
2. Add one cup of water (if you find the shake too thick add more water).
3. Blend all of the items and drink.
4. Toast one piece of bread and top it with one tbsp of almond butter.

Lunch: Grilled Salmon Salad

	Protein	Fat	Carbs	Calories	Fiber, total dietary
Tomatoes, red, ripe, raw, average, 2 medium whole (2 ⅗" dia.)	2	1	11	52	3
Cucumber (with peel), 1 cup, sliced	1	0	3	14	1
Romaine lettuce (salad), 2 cups, shredded	2	0	3	16	2
Balsamic vinegar, 2 tbsp	0	0	4	16	0
Atlantic salmon filet, 6 oz	43	14	0	309	0
Meal Totals	**48**	**15**	**21**	**407**	**6**

Directions:

1. Grill the salmon until it is opaque throughout and flakes easily with a fork.
2. Combine the lettuce and tomatoes in a bowl.
3. Top with the grilled salmon and drizzle with balsamic vinegar.

Dinner: Grilled Flank Steak with Broccoli

	Protein	Fat	Carbs	Calories	Fiber, total dietary
Broccoli, fresh, 15 spears (about 5" long)	14	2	24	130	14
Flank steak, 5 oz	29	11	0	218	0
Brown rice, medium grain, ¾ cup	3	1	34	164	3
Meal Totals	**46**	**14**	**58**	**512**	**17**

Directions:

1. Grill the steak until done to your liking (approximately 4-5 minutes a side).
2. Steam the broccoli spears and cook the brown rice until done.

Snack 1: Turkey Lettuce Wraps
Snack 2: Greek Yogurt

Turkey breast meat, 4 slices	15	1	4	88	0
Romaine lettuce (salad), 4 inner leaves	1	0	1	6	1
Fage - 0%, 8 oz	20	0	9	120	0
Meal Totals	**36**	**1**	**14**	**214**	**1**
Daily Totals	**163**	**43**	**154**	**1603**	**36**

Day 7

Breakfast: Greek Yogurt with Fresh Fruit

	Protein	Fat	Carbs	Calories	Fiber, total dietary
Blueberries, fresh, 30	0	0	6	23	1
Kiwi fruit, 1 fruit without skin, large	1	0	14	56	3
Strawberries, fresh, 20 medium (1 ¼" dia.)	1	1	17	72	6
Almonds, 6	2	4	1	42	1
Flaxseed, 1 tbsp	2	4	4	59	3
Fage - 0%, 8 oz	20	0	9	120	0
Meal Totals	**26**	**9**	**51**	**372**	**14**

Directions:

1. Scoop the Greek yogurt into a bowl.
2. Stir in the flaxseeds and top with blueberries, kiwi, strawberries, and almonds.

Lunch: Hummus Chicken Wrap

	Protein	Fat	Carbs	Calories	Fiber, total dietary
Hummus, ¼ cup	5	6	9	104	4
La Tortilla Factory Low-Carb Tortilla, 1 serving	5	2	10	50	7
Peppers, sweet, green, fresh, ½ large (2 ¼ per lb, approx 3 ¾" long, 3" dia.)	1	0	5	22	1
Chicken breast, no skin, 4 oz	26	1	0	125	0
Meal Totals	**37**	**9**	**24**	**301**	**12**

Directions:

1. Grill the chicken breast and slice it.
2. Take the tortilla and spread the hummus evenly over it.
3. Add the sliced chicken and sliced peppers and fold it into a wrap.

Dinner: Grilled Chicken and Fresh Salsa

	Protein	Fat	Carbs	Calories	Fiber, total dietary
Lime juice, 1 lime yield	0	0	3	10	0
Chicken breast, no skin, 4 oz	27	1	0	130	0
Sweet corn, fresh, ¼ cup	1	0	7	33	1
Onions, raw, ¼ cup, chopped	0	0	3	15	1
Cilantro, raw, 3 tbsp	0	0	0	0	0
Beans, black, ¼ cup	4	0	10	57	4
Jalapeño pepper, 1	0	0	1	4	0
Tomatoes, red, ripe, raw, average, 1 ½ cups, chopped or sliced	2	1	13	57	3
Meal Totals	**34**	**2**	**37**	**306**	**9**

Directions:

1. Mix the corn, diced onion, diced tomatoes, cilantro, black beans, and diced jalapeño in a bowl (for extra spice, leave the seeds in; for less heat, remove the seeds).
2. Squeeze the fresh lime over the mixture and stir.
3. Grill the chicken and top with the fresh salsa.

Snack: Cucumber with Hummus

Hummus, ¼ cup	5	6	9	104	4
Cucumber (with peel), 1 cup, sliced	1	0	3	14	1
Meal Totals	**6**	**6**	**12**	**118**	**5**
Daily Totals	**103**	**26**	**124**	**1097**	**40**

Day 8

Breakfast: Open-Face Banana-Almond-Butter Sandwich

	Protein	Fat	Carbs	Calories	Fiber, total dietary
Banana, fresh, 1 small (6" to 6 7/8" long)	1	1	24	93	2
Almond butter, 1 1/2 tbsp	4	14	5	152	1
Ezekiel 4:9 Sprouted Grain Bread (1 slice), 2 servings	8	1	30	160	6
Meal Totals	**13**	**16**	**59**	**405**	**9**

Directions:

1. Toast the bread and spread almond butter evenly over it.
2. Slice the banana and place the slices on top of the almond butter.

Lunch: Salad with Grilled Tuna

	Protein	Fat	Carbs	Calories	Fiber, total dietary
Balsamic vinegar, 2 tbsp	0	0	4	16	0
Red, ripe tomatoes, 1 cup cherry tomatoes	1	0	7	31	2
Yellow fin tuna filet, 4 oz	34	1	0	158	0
Snap peas, 1 cup	2	0	5	28	2
Olive oil, 1 tsp	0	5	0	40	0
Carrots, raw, 10 strips, medium	0	0	4	16	1
Romaine lettuce (salad), 1 1/2 cups, shredded	1	0	2	12	1
Meal Totals	**38**	**6**	**22**	**301**	**6**

Directions:

1. Grill the tuna to your liking.
2. Combine the lettuce, snap peas, tomato, and carrots in a bowl and top with the grilled tuna.
3. In a separate bowl, whisk together the balsamic vinegar and the olive oil.
4. Drizzle the balsamic vinaigrette over the salad.

Dinner: Chicken Stew

	Protein	Fat	Carbs	Calories	Fiber, total dietary
Mushrooms, fresh, ¾ cup, pieces or slices	2	0	2	12	1
Carrots, raw, ½ cup, chopped	1	0	6	26	2
Garlic, 1 clove	0	0	1	4	0
Onions, raw, ½ cup, chopped	1	0	7	30	1
Green peppers (bell peppers), ¾ cup, strips	1	0	7	28	1
Chicken breast, no skin, 4 oz	26	1	0	140	0
Pepper, black, 1 tbsp	1	0	4	16	2
Campbell's low-sodium chicken broth, 2 cups	6	0	2	26	0
White wine, 2 oz	0	0	0	40	0
Meal Totals	**38**	**1**	**29**	**322**	**7**

Directions:

1. Cook the chicken until done.
2. Add cooked chicken, mushrooms, carrots, chopped garlic, chopped onions, chopped green peppers in a medium saucepan.
3. Add two cups of chicken broth, black pepper, and white wine and let it simmer for 15 to 25 minutes.

Snack: Almonds

Almonds, 15	4	9	4	104	2
Meal Totals	**4**	**9**	**4**	**104**	**2**
Daily Totals	**93**	**32**	**113**	**1117**	**24**

Day 9

Breakfast: Super Oatmeal with Fresh Fruit

	Protein	Fat	Carbs	Calories	Fiber, total dietary
Raspberries, 30	1	O	7	28	4
Blueberries, fresh, 30	O	O	6	23	1
Oats, ¾ cup	7	4	78	225	12
On Gold Standard 100% Whey Protein, 2 servings	48	2	6	240	O
Meal Totals	**56**	**6**	**97**	**516**	**17**

Directions:

1. Cook oats until done.
2. Place the oats in a bowl and stir in the protein powder until dissolved.
3. Add a little water if needed to make it easy to stir in.

Lunch: Grilled Chicken Salad

	Protein	Fat	Carbs	Calories	Fiber, total dietary
Arugula, 4 cups	2	1	3	20	1
Balsamic vinegar, 2 tbsp	0	0	4	16	0
Onions, raw, ½ cup, chopped	1	0	7	30	1
Tomato, red, ripe, raw, average, 1 medium whole (2 ⅗" dia.)	1	0	6	26	1
Chicken breast, no skin, 4 oz	26	1	0	140	0
Avocado, California (Haas), ½ fruit without skin and seed	2	13	7	144	6
Carrots, raw, ½ cup, strips or slices	1	0	6	25	2
Cucumber (with peel), 1 cup, sliced	1	0	3	14	1
Radishes, 1 cup, sliced	1	0	4	19	2
Meal Totals	**35**	**15**	**40**	**434**	**14**

Directions:

1. Grill the chicken and slice.
2. Place arugula, chopped onions, tomatoes, carrots, cucumbers, radishes, and sliced avocado in a bowl.
3. Top with grilled chicken and drizzle with balsamic vinegar.

Dinner: Chicken with Sautéed Vegetables

	Protein	Fat	Carbs	Calories	Fiber, total dietary
Peppers, sweet, red, fresh, ½ cup, sliced	0	0	3	12	1
Olive oil, 1 tbsp	0	14	0	119	0
Chicken breast, no skin, 7 oz	54	3	0	245	0
Green peppers (bell peppers), ½ cup, chopped	1	0	5	19	1
Onions, raw, ¼ cup, sliced	0	0	2	11	1
Meal Totals	**55**	**17**	**10**	**406**	**3**

Directions:
1. Coat the inside of a nonstick skillet with cooking spray and cook chicken until fully cooked.
2. Remove chicken from pan and add olive oil, green and red peppers, and onions.
3. Cook in pan for 5-7 minutes or until tender.

Snack 1: Almonds
Snack 2: Dried Cranberries

Almonds, 15	4	9	4	104	2
Cranberries, dried, sweetened (craisins), ¼ cup	0	0	25	93	2
Meal Totals	**4**	**9**	**29**	**197**	**4**
Daily Totals	**150**	**47**	**176**	**1553**	**38**

Day 10

Breakfast: Eggs with Peppers and Mushrooms

	Protein	Fat	Carbs	Calories	Fiber, total dietary
Egg white, 5 servings	25	1	1	85	0
Green peppers (bell peppers), 1 cup, strips	1	0	9	38	2
Ezekiel 4:9 Sprouted Grain Bread (1 slice), 1 serving	4	1	15	80	3
Cottage cheese, 2% milk fat, ½ cup (not packed)	14	1	3	81	0
Avocado, California (Haas), ¼ fruit without skin and seed	1	7	4	72	3
Mushrooms, fresh, 1 cup, pieces or slices	2	0	2	15	1
Onions, raw, ½ cup, chopped	1	0	7	30	1
Meal Totals	**48**	**10**	**41**	**401**	**10**

Directions:

1. Coat the inside of a nonstick skillet with cooking spray.
2. Mix the egg whites, peppers, mushrooms, and onions in a bowl and add to the pan.
3. Scramble until fully cooked. Slice the avocado and place on top of the cooked eggs.
4. Toast the bread and serve the cottage cheese on the side.

Lunch: Grilled Chicken Spinach Salad

	Protein	Fat	Carbs	Calories	Fiber, total dietary
Cucumber (with peel), 1 cucumber (8 ¼")	2	0	8	39	2
Chicken breast, no skin, 4 oz	26	1	0	140	0
Spinach, fresh, 3 cups	3	0	3	21	2
Tomato, red, ripe, raw, average, 1 medium whole (2 ⅗" dia.)	1	0	6	26	1
Balsamic vinegar, 4 tbsp	0	0	8	32	0
Pine nuts, 30	1	4	1	36	0
Meal Totals	**33**	**5**	**26**	**294**	**5**

Directions:

1. Grill the chicken and slice.
2. Combine the spinach, sliced cucumber, tomatoes, and pine nuts in a bowl.
3. Top with grilled chicken and drizzle with the balsamic vinegar.

Dinner: Poached or Grilled Salmon

	Protein	Fat	Carbs	Calories	Fiber, total dietary
Asparagus, fresh, 15 spears, medium (5 ¼" to 7" long)	5	0	11	55	5
Sesame seeds, ½ tbsp	1	2	1	26	1
Atlantic salmon filet, 3 oz	22	7	0	155	0
Brown rice, medium grain, ½ cup	2	1	23	109	2
Meal Totals	**30**	**10**	**35**	**345**	**8**

Directions:
1. Place the salmon in an 8" x 8" baking dish.
2. Sprinkle with sesame seeds.
3. Add water to dish.
4. Cover and cook in the microwave on high for 8 minutes or until the fish turns opaque throughout and flakes easily when tested with a fork.
5. Alternatively, grill the fish.
6. Steam the asparagus and cook the brown rice and serve with the salmon.

Snack: Wheat Bran Muffin

Wheat bran muffin, 1, toasted	2	3	19	106	3
Meal Totals	**2**	**3**	**19**	**106**	**3**
Daily Totals	**113**	**28**	**121**	**1131**	**26**

Day 11

Breakfast: Protein Cottage Cheese with Fresh Fruit

	Protein	Fat	Carbs	Calories	Fiber, total dietary
Cottage cheese, 2%, 1 cup	24	10	12	240	0
On Gold Standard 100% Whey Protein, ¾ serving	18	1	2	90	0
Kiwi fruit, 1 fruit without skin, large	1	0	14	56	3
Raspberries, 30	1	0	7	28	4
Meal Totals	**44**	**11**	**35**	**414**	**7**

Directions:

1. Place the cottage cheese in a bowl and stir in the protein powder.
2. Top with the kiwi and raspberries.

Lunch: Shrimp Salad

	Protein	Fat	Carbs	Calories	Fiber, total dietary
French salad dressing, low fat, 2 tbsp	0	2	7	44	0
Tossed salad, 1 ½ cups	3	0	7	33	0
Shrimp, cooked, 4 oz	24	1	0	112	0
Chickpeas (garbanzo beans), ¼ cup	3	1	14	71	3
Peppers, sweet, red, fresh, 1 cup, sliced	1	0	6	25	2
Onions, raw, 4 slices, thin	0	0	3	14	1
Green peppers (bell peppers), 1 cup, strips	1	0	9	38	2
Meal Totals	**32**	**4**	**46**	**337**	**8**

Directions:

1. Coat the inside of a nonstick skillet with cooking spray and place shrimp into pan.
2. Cook until pink and cooked throughout.
3. Combine salad, cooked shrimp, chickpeas, green and red peppers, onions.
4. Drizzle with French salad dressing.

Dinner: Spicy Chicken Stir-Fry

	Protein	Fat	Carbs	Calories	Fiber, total dietary
Sriracha chili sauce, 2 tsp	0	0	2	10	0
Chicken breast, no skin, 4 oz	26	1	0	140	0
Asparagus, fresh, 15 spears, medium (5 ¼" to 7" long)	5	0	11	55	5
Garlic, 2 cloves	0	0	2	9	0
Ginger root, 5 slices (1" dia.)	0	0	2	9	0
Mushrooms, fresh, 1 cup, pieces or slices	2	0	2	15	1
Brown rice, medium grain, ¼ cup	1	0	11	55	1
Meal Totals	**34**	**1**	**30**	**293**	**7**

Directions:

1. Coat the inside of a nonstick skillet with cooking spray and cook chicken until fully cooked throughout.
2. Remove chicken from pan and slice.
3. Re-spray pan and add sliced asparagus, sliced ginger, sliced garlic, and mushrooms.
4. Sauté for 5–7 minutes.
5. Add cooked chicken and stir in Sriracha chili sauce.
6. Serve stir-fry on a bed of cooked brown rice.

Snack: Almonds

Almonds, 15	4	9	4	104	2
Meal Totals	**4**	**9**	**4**	**104**	**2**
Daily Totals	**114**	**25**	**116**	**1133**	**24**

Day 12

Breakfast: Egg White Scramble

	Protein	Fat	Carbs	Calories	Fiber, total dietary
Egg white, fresh, 5 large	20	0	0	85	0
Ezekiel 4:9 Sprouted Grain Bread (1 slice), 2 servings	8	1	30	160	6
Louis Rich Turkey Bacon (1 slice), 3 servings	6	7	0	105	0
Almond butter, ½ tbsp	1	5	2	51	0
Cheddar or colby cheese, low fat, 2 slices (1 oz)	14	4	1	98	0
Meal Totals	**49**	**17**	**33**	**499**	**6**

Directions:

1. Coat the inside of a nonstick skillet with cooking spray.
2. Mix the egg whites and cooked turkey bacon in a bowl and add to the pan.
3. Scramble until fully cooked and top with cheese.
4. Toast the bread and evenly spread the almond butter on top.

Lunch: Turkey Wrap

	Protein	Fat	Carbs	Calories	Fiber, total dietary
Cheddar or colby cheese, low fat, 1 slice (1 oz)	7	2	1	49	0
Turkey breast meat, 3 slices	11	1	3	66	0
Beans, black, 1 cup	15	1	41	227	15
La Tortilla Factory Low-Carb Tortilla, 1 serving	5	2	10	50	7
Meal Totals	**38**	**6**	**55**	**392**	**22**

Directions:

1. Place the cheese slice, turkey, and black beans in the tortilla.
2. Fold the tortilla into a wrap.
3. For some extra spice, add a little Sriracha hot chili sauce.

Dinner: Stewed Chicken over Rice

	Protein	Fat	Carbs	Calories	Fiber, total dietary
Campbell's low-sodium chicken broth, 1 cup	3	0	1	13	0
Tomato, red, ripe, raw, average, 1 medium whole (2 3/5" dia.)	1	0	6	26	1
Brown rice, medium grain, 3/4 cup	3	1	34	164	3
Garlic, 3 cloves	1	0	3	13	0
Onions, raw, 1/2 cup, chopped	1	0	7	30	1
Parsley, 10 sprigs	0	0	1	4	0
Chicken breast, no skin, 7 oz	54	3	0	245	0
Meal Totals	**63**	**5**	**51**	**495**	**6**

Directions:
1. Cook chicken and slice.
2. In a medium saucepan, add cooked chicken, chicken broth, tomatoes, sliced garlic, onions, and chopped parsley.
3. Bring to a boil and reduce heat and let it simmer for 20–25 minutes or until most liquid is gone.
4. Serve over cooked brown rice.

Snack 1: Milk
Snack 2: Almonds

Milk, 1%, 1 cup	8	2	12	110	0
Almonds, 15	4	9	4	104	2
Meal Totals	**12**	**11**	**16**	**214**	**2**
Daily Totals	**162**	**39**	**155**	**1615**	**36**

Day 13

Breakfast: Cereal with Fresh Fruit

	Protein	Fat	Carbs	Calories	Fiber, total dietary
Milk, 1%, ¾ cup	6	2	9	83	0
Fiber One cereal, 1 cup (1 serving)	4	2	50	120	28
Flaxseed, 1 tbsp	2	4	4	59	3
Blueberries, fresh, 1 cup	1	0	21	81	4
Strawberries, fresh, 10 medium (1 ¼" dia.)	1	0	8	36	3
Meal Totals	**14**	**8**	**92**	**379**	**38**

Directions:

1. Add cereal and milk to a bowl.
2. Place the blueberries, strawberries, and flaxseed on top of the cereal.

Lunch: Chicken Breast Wrap

	Protein	Fat	Carbs	Calories	Fiber, total dietary
Alfalfa sprouts, 2 cups	3	0	2	19	2
Tomato, red, ripe, raw, average, 1 medium whole (2 3/5" dia.)	1	0	6	26	1
La Tortilla Factory Whole Wheat Low-Carb Tortilla, 1 serving	5	2	10	50	7
Tzatziki dip, 3 tbsp	2	6	3	75	0
Chicken breast, no skin, 4 oz	26	1	0	140	0
Meal Totals	**37**	**9**	**21**	**310**	**10**

Directions:

1. Take the tortilla and spread the tzatziki dip over it.
2. Add the sliced tomatoes, alfalfa sprouts, and cooked chicken.

Dinner: Dill Salmon with Steamed Vegetables

	Protein	Fat	Carbs	Calories	Fiber, total dietary
Dill weed, fresh, 5 sprigs	0	0	0	0	0
Summer squash, ½ cup, sliced	1	0	2	9	1
Atlantic salmon filet, 5 oz	36	12	0	258	0
Lemon, ½ fruit without seeds	1	0	6	11	3
Onions, raw, ¼ cup, chopped	0	0	3	15	1
Zucchini, ½ cup, sliced	1	0	4	14	1
Meal Totals	**39**	**12**	**15**	**307**	**6**

Directions:

1. Coat the inside of a nonstick pan with spray; turn it on to medium heat.
2. Cook until salmon easily flakes with a fork and top with dill.
3. Sprinkle with lemon juice.
4. Dice the summer squash, onions, and zucchini and steam and serve on the side of the salmon.

Snack: String Cheese

Laughing Cow Original Cheese, 2 servings	4	8	2	100	0
Meal Totals	**4**	**8**	**2**	**100**	**0**
Daily Totals	**94**	**37**	**130**	**1081**	**54**

Day 14

Breakfast: Fresh Fruit and Toast

	Protein	Fat	Carbs	Calories	Fiber, total dietary
Strawberries, fresh, 15 medium (1 ¼" dia.)	1	1	13	54	4
Ezekiel 4:9 Sprouted Grain Bread (1 slice), 2 servings	8	1	30	160	6
Almond butter, 1 tbsp	2	9	3	101	1
Apple, fresh, 1 medium (2 ¾" dia.) (approx 3 per lb)	0	0	21	81	4
Meal Totals	**11**	**11**	**67**	**396**	**15**

Directions:

1. Slice strawberries and apples and place in a bowl.
2. Toast the bread and evenly spread the almond butter on the bread.

Lunch: Taco Salad

	Protein	Fat	Carbs	Calories	Fiber, total dietary
Chicken breast, no skin, 4 oz	26	1	0	140	0
Salsa, ½ cup	2	0	8	36	2
Chili powder, 1 tsp	0	0	1	8	1
Garlic powder, 1 tsp	0	0	2	9	0
Romaine lettuce (salad), 3 cups, shredded	3	0	4	24	3
Green peppers (bell peppers), 1 cup, strips	1	0	9	38	2
Karas Egg, 1 serving	6	7	1	90	0
Meal Totals	**38**	**8**	**25**	**345**	**8**

Directions:
1. Season the chicken with chili powder and garlic powder.
2. Cook and slice the chicken.
3. Combine the lettuce with green peppers, hard-boiled egg, and cooked chicken and top with salsa.

Dinner: Shrimp Stir-Fry

	Protein	Fat	Carbs	Calories	Fiber, total dietary
Green peppers (bell peppers), 1 cup, strips	1	0	9	38	2
Scallions, raw, 1 medium (4 1/8" long)	0	0	1	5	0
Lemon, 1/2 fruit without seeds	1	0	6	11	3
Hot chili pepper, 1	1	0	4	18	1
Peppers, sweet, red, fresh, 1 cup, chopped	1	0	10	40	3
Shrimp, raw, 30 medium	37	3	2	191	0
Meal Totals	**41**	**3**	**32**	**303**	**9**

Directions:

1. Coat the inside of a nonstick skillet with cooking spray.
2. Add shrimp, green and red peppers, sliced scallions, and sliced chili peppers.
3. Sauté for 10-12 minutes or until all items are fully cooked.
4. Drizzle with lemon juice.

Snack: Almonds

Almonds, 15	4	9	4	104	2
Meal Totals	**4**	**9**	**4**	**104**	**2**
Daily Totals	**94**	**31**	**128**	**1133**	**34**

Day 15

Breakfast: Open-Face Egg Sandwich

	Protein	Fat	Carbs	Calories	Fiber, total dietary
Tomatoes, red, ripe, raw, average, 2 medium whole (2 ⅗" dia.)	2	1	11	52	3
Ezekiel 4:9 Sprouted Grain Bread (1 slice), 1 serving	4	1	15	80	3
Spinach, fresh, 4 cups	3	0	4	28	3
Karas Egg, 2 servings	13	14	2	180	0
Cottage cheese, 2%, ½ cup	12	5	6	120	0
Olive oil, 1 tsp	0	5	0	40	0
Meal Totals	**34**	**26**	**38**	**500**	**9**

Directions:
1. Coat the inside of a nonstick skillet with cooking spray.
2. Cook eggs and place on top of toast with sliced tomatoes.
3. Sauté the spinach in olive oil and place it on top of eggs and tomatoes.
4. Serve cottage cheese on the side.

Lunch: Turkey Sandwich

	Protein	Fat	Carbs	Calories	Fiber, total dietary
Turkey breast meat, 4 slices	15	1	4	88	0
Grey Poupon de Dijon mustard, 1 tsp	0	0	0	5	0
Philadelphia Herb & Garlic Cream Cheese, 2 tbsp	2	8	2	90	0
Cucumber (peeled), 8 slices	0	0	1	7	0
Ezekiel 4:9 Sprouted Grain Bread (1 slice), 2 servings	8	1	30	160	6
Tomato, red, ripe, raw, average, 3 slices, medium (¼" thick)	1	0	3	13	1
Meal Totals	**26**	**10**	**40**	**363**	**7**

Directions:

1. Toast bread and spread with the mustard and cream cheese.
2. Add the turkey, sliced cucumbers, and tomatoes to the sandwich.

Dinner: Mahimahi over Rice

	Protein	Fat	Carbs	Calories	Fiber, total dietary
Garlic, 3 cloves	1	0	3	13	0
Broccoli, fresh, 2 cups, chopped	5	1	9	49	5
Onions, raw, ¼ cup, chopped	0	0	3	15	1
Cilantro, raw, 4 tbsp	0	0	0	0	0
Mahimahi, 6 oz	40	2	0	180	0
Brown rice, medium grain, 1 cup	5	2	46	218	4
Olive oil, ½ tbsp	0	7	0	60	0
Meal Totals	**51**	**12**	**61**	**535**	**10**

Directions:

1. Coat the inside of a nonstick skillet with olive oil.
2. Cook mahimahi until it is opaque throughout and easily flakes with a fork.
3. Top the fish with chopped cilantro and sautéed onions.
4. Steam the broccoli with chopped garlic and serve the fish on a bed of cooked brown rice.

Snack 1: Apple
Snack 2: Greek Yogurt

	Protein	Fat	Carbs	Calories	Fiber, total dietary
Apple, fresh, 1 medium (2 ¾" dia.) (approx 3 per lb)	0	0	21	81	4
Oikos Organic Greek Yogurt, plain, 6 oz	15	0	6	80	0
Raspberries, 20	0	0	4	19	3
Meal Totals	**15**	**0**	**31**	**180**	**7**
Daily Totals	**126**	**48**	**170**	**1578**	**32**

Day 16

Breakfast: Mexican Egg Scramble

	Protein	Fat	Carbs	Calories	Fiber, total dietary
Onions, raw, 1 cup, chopped	2	0	14	61	3
Jalapeño peppers, 2	0	0	2	8	1
Beans, black, ¼ cup	4	0	10	57	4
Egg white, 4 servings	20	0	1	68	0
Avocado, California (Haas), ⅖ fruit without skin and seed	1	11	6	116	5
Salsa, 1 cup	3	1	16	73	4
Meal Totals	**30**	**12**	**49**	**383**	**17**

Directions:

1. Coat the inside of a nonstick skillet with cooking spray.
2. Mix the egg whites, jalapeños, black beans, and onions in a bowl and add to the pan.
3. Scramble until fully cooked.
4. Slice the avocado and place on top of the cooked eggs.
5. Place salsa over the scramble.

Lunch: Spicy Tuna Sandwich

	Protein	Fat	Carbs	Calories	Fiber, total dietary
Kraft Fat-Free Mayonnaise or Salad Dressing, 2 tbsp	0	1	4	22	1
Sriracha chili sauce, 1 tsp	0	0	1	5	0
Tuna, Starkist Chunk White Albacore in Water, 2 ½ servings	33	5	0	175	0
Ezekiel 4:9 Sprouted Grain Bread (1 slice), 1 serving	4	1	15	80	3
Celery, raw, 1 stalk, large (11"–12" long)	0	0	2	10	1
Meal Totals	**37**	**7**	**22**	**292**	**5**

Directions:

1. Open and drain the tuna and place it in a bowl.
2. Stir in mayo, Sriracha chili sauce, and chopped celery.
3. Place contents of the bowl on toasted bread.

Dinner: Teriyaki Pork Tenderloin Salad

	Protein	Fat	Carbs	Calories	Fiber, total dietary
Romaine lettuce (salad), ½ cup, shredded	0	0	1	4	0
Onions, raw, ¼ cup, chopped	0	0	3	15	1
Balsamic vinegar, 1 tbsp	0	0	2	8	0
Teriyaki sauce (1 tbsp), 1 packet	1	0	3	16	0
Pork tenderloin, 4 oz	33	9	0	228	3
Beet, fresh, 1 (2" dia.)	1	0	8	35	2
Meal Totals	**35**	**9**	**17**	**306**	**6**

Directions:

1. Place pork tenderloin in 8" x 8" baking dish and top with teriyaki sauce.
2. Bake at 350 degrees for 35-45 minutes.
3. Combine the lettuce, onions, beets, cooked pork tenderloin.
4. Drizzle with balsamic vinegar.

Snack: Apple with Almond Butter

Apple, fresh, 1 small (2 ½" dia.) (approx 4 per lb)	0	0	16	63	3
Almond butter, ½ tbsp	1	5	2	51	0
Meal Totals	**1**	**5**	**18**	**114**	**3**
Daily Totals	**103**	**33**	**106**	**1095**	**31**

Day 17

Breakfast: Cereal with Fresh Fruit and Toast

	Protein	Fat	Carbs	Calories	Fiber, total dietary
Ezekiel 4:9 Sprouted Grain Bread (1 slice), 1 serving	4	1	15	80	3
Fiber One cereal, ½ cup (1 serving)	2	1	25	60	14
Blueberries, fresh, 1 cup	1	0	21	81	4
Strawberries, fresh, 1 cup, halves	1	1	11	46	4
Milk, 1%, 1 cup	8	2	12	110	0
Meal Totals	**16**	**5**	**84**	**377**	**25**

Directions:

1. Place milk and cereal in a bowl.
2. Top with blueberries, strawberries.
3. Serve with a side of toast.

Lunch: Ground Turkey with Peppers and Onions

	Protein	Fat	Carbs	Calories	Fiber, total dietary
Peppers, sweet, red, fresh, 1 large (2 ¼ per lb, approx 3 ¾" long, 3" dia.)	1	0	11	44	3
Ground turkey, 1 patty (4 oz, raw, yield after cooking)	22	11	0	193	0
Onions, raw, ¼ cup, chopped	0	0	3	15	1
Garlic, 3 cloves	1	0	3	13	0
Basil, 5 leaves	0	0	0	1	0
Parmesan cheese, grated, 1 ½ tbsp	3	2	0	34	0
Meal Totals	**27**	**13**	**17**	**300**	**4**

Directions:

1. Coat the inside of a nonstick skillet with cooking spray.
2. Add the ground turkey and cook until fully cooked.
3. Add the peppers, onions, chopped garlic, and basil.
4. Cook on medium for 5-7 minutes.
5. Sprinkle with Parmesan cheese.

Dinner: Pan-Seared Mahimahi with Vegetables

	Protein	Fat	Carbs	Calories	Fiber, total dietary
Brussels sprouts, cooked, 10	5	1	15	76	5
Almonds, ⅕ cup, slivered	5	11	4	125	3
Mahimahi, 4 oz	27	1	0	120	0
Scallions, raw, 1 medium (4 ⅛" long)	0	0	1	5	0
Meal Totals	**37**	**13**	**20**	**326**	**8**

Directions:

1. Coat the inside of a nonstick skillet with cooking spray.
2. Cook mahimahi until it is opaque throughout and easily flakes with a fork.
3. For some extra heat, sprinkle some red chili flakes on top of the fish.
4. Steam brussels sprouts with slivered almonds and serve on the side.

Snack: Greek Yogurt

Fage – 0%, 8 oz	20	0	9	120	0
Meal Totals	**20**	**0**	**9**	**120**	**0**
Daily Totals	**100**	**31**	**130**	**1123**	**37**

Day 18

Breakfast: Oatmeal and Eggs

	Protein	Fat	Carbs	Calories	Fiber, total dietary
Cinnamon, ground, 1 tbsp	0	0	5	18	4
Strawberries, fresh, 6 medium (1 ¼" dia.)	0	0	5	22	2
Egg white, 4 servings	20	0	1	68	0
Cottage cheese, 2%, ¾ cup	18	8	9	180	0
Oats, ⅖ cup	4	2	41	120	7
Karas Egg, 1 serving	6	7	1	90	0
Meal Totals	**48**	**17**	**62**	**498**	**13**

Directions:

1. Cook oats until done, stir in cinnamon, and top with strawberries.
2. Coat the inside of a nonstick skillet with cooking spray.
3. Mix the egg whites and one egg together.
4. Scramble until fully cooked and serve cottage cheese on the side.

Lunch: Chickpea and Spinach Salad

	Protein	Fat	Carbs	Calories	Fiber, total dietary
Chickpeas, ½ cup	7	2	23	135	6
Balsamic vinegar, 2 tbsp	0	0	4	16	0
Spinach, fresh, 3 cups	3	0	3	21	2
Tomato, red, ripe, raw, average, 1 medium whole (2 ⅗" dia.)	1	0	6	26	1
Carrots, raw, ½ cup, strips or slices	1	0	6	25	2
Cucumber (peeled), 1 cup, sliced	1	0	3	14	1
Olive oil, 1 tsp	0	5	0	40	0
Goat cheese, soft, 2 oz	11	12	1	152	0
Meal Totals	**24**	**19**	**46**	**429**	**12**

Directions:

1. Combine the spinach, chickpeas, tomatoes, carrots, cucumbers, and goat cheese in a bowl.
2. In a separate bowl, whisk together the balsamic vinegar and the olive oil.
3. Drizzle the balsamic vinaigrette over the salad.

Dinner: Tofu Stir-Fry

	Protein	Fat	Carbs	Calories	Fiber, total dietary
Broccoli, fresh, 2 cups, chopped	5	1	9	49	5
Lime juice, 3-wedge yield	0	0	1	4	0
Mushrooms, fresh, 2 ½ cups, pieces or slices	5	1	6	39	2
Soy sauce made from soy and wheat (shoyu), low sodium, 2 tbsp	2	0	3	19	0
Tofu, firm, ½ block	26	14	7	129	4
Bean sprouts, 1 cup	3	0	7	34	2
Brown rice, medium grain, ½ cup	2	1	23	109	2
Green peppers (bell peppers), 1 cup, strips	1	0	9	38	2
Meal Totals	**44**	**17**	**65**	**421**	**17**

Directions:

1. Coat the inside of a nonstick skillet with cooking spray and add broccoli, mushrooms, sliced tofu, bean sprouts, and green peppers.
2. Cook for 7–10 minutes.
3. Serve over a bed of brown rice and drizzle soy sauce over the top.

Snack 1: Greek Yogurt
Snack 2: Milk

Fage – 0%, 8 oz	20	0	9	120	0
Milk, 1%, 1 cup	8	2	12	110	0
Meal Totals	**28**	**2**	**21**	**230**	**0**
Daily Totals	**144**	**55**	**194**	**1578**	**42**

Day 19

Breakfast: Fresh Fruit Protein Shake with Bran Muffin

	Protein	Fat	Carbs	Calories	Fiber, total dietary
Milk, 1%, 1 cup	8	2	12	110	0
Apple, fresh, 1 medium (2 ¾" dia.) (approx 3 per lb)	0	0	21	81	4
Blueberries, fresh, 20	0	0	4	15	1
Wheat bran muffin, 1, toasted	2	3	19	106	3
On Gold Standard 100% Whey Protein, 1 serving	24	1	3	120	0
Meal Totals	**34**	**6**	**59**	**432**	**8**

Directions:

1. In a blender, combine apples, blueberries, milk, and protein powder and blend until smooth.
2. Toast the wheat bran muffin and serve on the side.

Lunch: Grilled Tuna Salad

	Protein	Fat	Carbs	Calories	Fiber, total dietary
Yellow fin tuna filet, 4 oz	34	1	0	158	0
Red, ripe cherry tomatoes, 1 cup	1	0	7	31	2
Snap peas, 1 cup	2	0	5	28	2
Balsamic vinegar, 2 tbsp	0	0	4	16	0
Olive oil, 1 tsp	0	5	0	40	0
Romaine lettuce (salad), 1 ½ cups, shredded	1	0	2	12	1
Carrots, raw, 10 strips, medium	0	0	4	16	1
Meal Totals	**38**	**6**	**22**	**301**	**6**

Directions:

1. Grill the tuna to your liking.
2. Combine lettuce, tomatoes, snap peas, carrots, and grilled tuna in a bowl.
3. In a separate bowl, whisk together the balsamic vinegar and olive oil.
4. Drizzle the balsamic vinaigrette over the salad.

Dinner: Grilled or Poached Salmon

	Protein	Fat	Carbs	Calories	Fiber, total dietary
Eggplant, fresh, 2 cups, cubes	2	0	10	43	4
Basil, 5 leaves	0	0	0	1	0
Chickpeas, ¼ cup	4	1	12	68	3
Brown rice, medium grain, ¼ cup	1	0	11	55	1
Atlantic salmon filet, 3 oz	22	7	0	155	0
Meal Totals	**29**	**8**	**33**	**322**	**8**

Directions:

1. Place the salmon in an 8" x 8" baking dish.
2. Add water to dish.
3. Cover and cook in the microwave on high for 8 minutes or until the fish turns opaque throughout and flakes easily when tested with a fork.
4. Alternatively, grill the fish.
5. Steam the eggplant and chickpeas with chopped basil and serve on the side.
6. Serve the salmon on a bed of cooked brown rice.

Snack: Almonds

Almonds, 15	4	9	4	104	2
Meal Totals	**4**	**9**	**4**	**104**	**2**
Daily Totals	**105**	**29**	**118**	**1159**	**24**

Day 20

Breakfast: Greek Yogurt with Fresh Fruit

	Protein	Fat	Carbs	Calories	Fiber, total dietary
Banana, fresh, 1 medium (7" to 7 7/8" long)	1	1	28	109	3
Blueberries, fresh, 25	0	0	5	19	1
Fage - 0%, 8 oz	20	0	9	120	0
Almond butter, 3/4 tbsp	2	7	3	76	0
Ezekiel 4:9 Sprouted Grain Bread (1 slice), 1 serving	4	1	15	80	3
Meal Totals	**27**	**9**	**60**	**404**	**7**

Directions:

1. Take the Greek yogurt and put it into a bowl.
2. On top of the yogurt, place sliced banana and blueberries.
3. Toast the bread and spread almond butter evenly over it.

Lunch: Cobb Salad

	Protein	Fat	Carbs	Calories	Fiber, total dietary
Balsamic vinegar, 2 tbsp	0	0	4	16	0
Spinach, fresh, 3 cups	3	0	3	21	2
Tomatoes, red, ripe, raw, average, 1 medium whole (2 3/5" dia.)	1	0	6	26	1
Louis Rich Turkey Bacon (1 slice), 3 servings	6	7	0	105	0
Cucumber (with peel), 1 cup, sliced	1	0	3	14	1
Chicken breast, no skin, 4 oz	26	1	0	140	0
Meal Totals	**37**	**8**	**16**	**322**	**4**

Directions:

1. Cook the chicken and slice.
2. Combine spinach, tomatoes, cooked turkey bacon, and cucumbers in a bowl.
3. Top with the cooked chicken and drizzle with the balsamic vinegar.

Dinner: Skirt Steak with Sautéed Vegetables

	Protein	Fat	Carbs.	Calories	Fiber, total dietary
Beef, skirt steak, lean, 4 oz	31	12	0	233	0
Tomato, red, ripe, raw, average, 4 slices, medium (1/4" thick)	1	0	4	17	1
Mushrooms, fresh, 1 cup, pieces or slices	2	0	2	15	1
Onions, raw, 1/4 cup, chopped	0	0	3	15	1
Green beans (snap), 1 cup	2	0	8	34	4
Meal Totals	**36**	**12**	**17**	**314**	**7**

Directions:

1. Grill the steak until done to your liking (approximately 4-5 minutes a side).
2. Coat the inside of a nonstick skillet with cooking spray and sauté tomatoes, mushrooms, onions, and green beans for 5-7 minutes.
3. Serve on the side of the steak.

Snack: Milk

	Protein	Fat	Carbs.	Calories	Fiber, total dietary
Milk, 1%, 1 cup	8	2	12	122	0
Meal Totals	**8**	**2**	**12**	**122**	**0**
Daily Totals	**108**	**31**	**105**	**1146**	**17**

Day 21

Breakfast: Egg Sandwich and Fruit

	Protein	Fat	Carbs	Calories	Fiber, total dietary
Cantaloupe, ½ melon, medium (about 5" dia.)	2	1	23	97	2
Tomatoes, red, ripe, raw, average, 2 medium whole (2 ⅗" dia.)	2	1	11	52	3
Grey Poupon de Dijon mustard, 2 tsp	0	0	0	10	0
Ezekiel 4:9 Sprouted Grain Bread (1 slice), 2 servings	8	1	30	160	6
Karas Egg, 2 servings	13	14	2	180	0
Meal Totals	**25**	**17**	**66**	**499**	**11**

Directions:

1. Coat the inside of a nonstick skillet with cooking spray.
2. Cook eggs and place on top of the toast with sliced tomatoes and mustard.
3. Cut the cantaloupe and serve it on the side.

Lunch: Grilled Chicken Salad

	Protein	Fat	Carbs	Calories	Fiber, total dietary
Balsamic vinegar, 2 tbsp	0	0	4	16	0
Green peppers (bell peppers), 1 cup, strips	1	0	9	38	2
Beets, fresh, 3 (2" dia.)	4	0	24	106	7
Cucumber (with peel), 1 cup, sliced	1	0	3	14	1
Romaine lettuce (salad), 2 ½ cups, shredded	2	0	3	20	2
Chicken breast, no skin, 4 oz	26	1	0	140	0
Feta cheese, 1 oz	4	6	1	75	0
Meal Totals	**38**	**7**	**44**	**409**	**12**

Directions:

1. Grill the chicken and slice.
2. Combine the lettuce, green peppers, beets, cucumbers, and feta cheese in a bowl.
3. Top with cooked chicken and drizzle with balsamic vinegar.

Dinner: Steak Stir-Fry

	Protein	Fat	Carbs	Calories	Fiber, total dietary
Ginger root, 2 slices (1" dia.)	0	0	1	4	0
Broccoli, fresh, 15 spears (about 5" long)	14	2	24	130	14
Water chestnuts, Chinese, canned, solids and liquids, ½ cup slices	1	0	9	35	2
Flank steak, 5 oz	29	11	0	218	0
Soy sauce made from soy and wheat (shoyu), low-sodium, 1 tbsp	1	0	2	10	0
Brown rice, medium grain, ½ cup	2	1	23	109	2
Meal Totals	**47**	**14**	**59**	**506**	**18**

Directions:

1. Coat the inside of a nonstick skillet with cooking spray.
2. Slice steak into small strips and add to the pan and cook until cooked throughout.
3. Add sliced ginger root, broccoli, and water chestnuts to pan and cook for 6–8 minutes.
4. Serve on top of a bed of brown rice and drizzle with soy sauce.

Snack 1: Greek Yogurt
Snack 2: Milk

Fage – 0%, 8 oz	20	0	9	120	0
Milk, 1%, 1 cup	8	2	12	110	0
Meal Totals	**28**	**2**	**21**	**230**	**0**
Daily Totals	**138**	**40**	**190**	**1629**	**41**

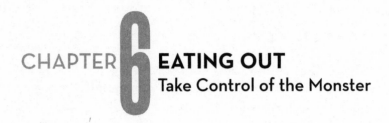

CHAPTER **6** **EATING OUT**
Take Control of the Monster

Yes. I call eating out "The Monster." Eating out has become an issue for *all* Americans, as the added fat and calories and the sheer size of most restaurant/fast-food portions are causing people of all sizes to gain weight. What constitutes a slight *storm* of calories for most people is a *tsunami* for Petites.

Managing Your Body Mass Index

Americans are eating out approximately five times a week, either at fast-food establishments or restaurants. This is critically important, as research shows that, for each additional meal eaten out, your body mass index (BMI) goes up. BMI is a number that is calculated simply by plugging your height and weight into an equation. Here is the equation:

Your Weight / Your Height in Inches Squared x 703 = Your BMI

To illustrate, I'm going to use my Petite from the introduction again. She was 5'3" and 170 pounds when she started. Her BMI equation would thus look like this:

$170 / 63^2 \times 703 = 30.11$.

If your BMI is between 18 and 24.9, you are considered at an acceptable weight. A BMI of 25 to 29.9 is considered overweight. A BMI of over 30 is considered obese.

So my client started out obese, which we both knew. But when she went down to 130 pounds, her goal weight (which she hit and stayed at), her BMI went down to 130 (her new weight) divided by her height squared (63 x 63) multiplied by 703 = 23. That 40-pound weight loss placed her in the acceptable range.

With just one meal eaten out a week, the research shows that a person's BMI will go up by one percentage point. That is how damaging restaurant eating can be to Petites, but it doesn't have to be. Why, you may ask, is eating out such as killer to your body weight? Read on.

The research from the Centers for Disease Control and Prevention regarding fruit and vegetable consumption showed that only 8 percent of Americans are eating the recommended two cups of fruit a day and only 6 percent are eating two and a half cups of vegetables a day.[1] What I didn't tell you was that food consumed outside the home constituted one-third of all calories eaten. But, when it comes to fruit and vegetable consumption, it only accounted for 11 percent of the calories they ate when eating out. If you do the math (and you know I *love* The Math), then 11 percent of one-third of the calories eaten out means that Americans are eating less than 3 percent of their calories from fruits and vegetables when eating out.

Let me repeat that—the average American is only eating 3 percent of their calories from fruits and vegetables when eating out.

That's terribly low. No, that's shockingly low, but it says a lot about what we are generally eating when eating out and why our BMI is going up with each meal eaten out. I'm going to help you reverse that trend when eating out and teach you how to eat many more tasty fruits and vegetables and stay full and satisfied, since they are the key to your success on this plan.

Here is even more research on calories when eating out to drive this point home. New York University dietitians, those educated and trained to look at the portion size and associated caloric value of foods, underestimated calories in restaurant food by 37 percent and fat content by 49 percent.[2] Yikes, that's worth repeating! Dietitians *underestimated* the total calories in each meal, on average, by 37 percent, and the fat content on average by 49 percent. Here are some of the discrepancies that occurred when it came to estimating calories and fat in each meal:

Food	Estimated Calories	Estimated Fat	Actual Cal & Fat
Hamburger and fries	863	44	1550 / 101
Tuna salad sandwich	374	18	720 / 43
Porterhouse steak dinner	1239	64	1860 / 125
Lasagna	694	35	960 / 53
Caesar salad	439	24	660 / 46

I took the time to show these numbers visually, as I wanted to emphasize the magnitude of this problem. A tall woman must realize that this is an issue. As a Petite, you have to see that the magnitude of the effect on your body is exponential. In one meal eaten out, you may possibly consume *all your calories* for the day. Any additional calories eaten that day will constitute "overflow" in your baby pool. By eating out, you get slammed with extra calories that you don't need, can't possibly burn off quickly, *and* probably don't even want. The reason that I keep repeating that you "probably don't even want" these calories is because that is a big part of the way I am going to teach you to eat when eating out. I will get rid of a lot of Addies and other ingredients in foods that add up to a lot of calories, but that truly don't add to the flavor that you desire.

What about the old recommendation "when eating out, eat in moderation"? Unfortunately, we have lost all semblance of what constitutes "moderation," as our portion sizes are huge and the foods that we are generally consuming when eating out are not what are best for our minds, bodies, and body weight. I've already shown that people are not eating fruits and vegetables when eating out. And, because of cost, you have to assume that the majority of what is eaten outside of the home is in the form of processed carbohydrates. I need to help you redefine "moderation" and make sure that you don't feel deprived at the same time. I'm not at all a fan of deprivation and all the research leads to the fact that deprivation will only lead to a binge. Remember, my goal is to manage your hunger.

Let me start by giving your general "eating-out" guidelines for breakfast, lunch, and dinner, then help you manage the menu in the most popular types of restaurants—steak houses, Italian, Mexican, Chinese, Thai, Greek, and sushi restaurants. I'm going to show you options for both your 1100-calorie days and for your 1600-calorie days.

Breakfast

Here is what I want you to order. These are 400-calorie approximations for breakfast options.

2 poached eggs	180 calories
1 piece of whole-wheat toast	100 calories
1 piece or cup of cut-up fruit	100 calories
Subtotal	**380 calories**

Or

1 cup of Fiber One cereal	120 calories
¾ cup 2% milk	102 calories
1 piece or cup of cut-up fruit	100 calories
Subtotal	**322 calories**

Or

oatmeal	225 calories
½ cup 2% milk	68 calories
1 piece or cup of cut-up fruit	100 calories
Subtotal	**393 calories**

For your 500-calorie breakfast days, add:

3 pieces of low-fat turkey bacon	105 calories

Or

a second piece/cup of fruit	100 calories

Or

1 tbsp of butter on your bread	80 calories

Or

2 tbsp of jam	100 calories

Here is what I want you to avoid when eating breakfast out: heavy carb items such as

- pancakes

- French toast

- waffles

- simple-carb cereals

Save these items for very special occasions and, even then, keep the portion size down. Sure, it would be better if the pancakes, French toast, and waffles were made with whole grains or whole wheat, but the sheer size of the portion plus the amount of butter and syrup generally adds up to a lot of calories. That's too much "spillage" in your baby-size pool.

Once you have completed your first twenty-one days on my plan, here is an option for breakfast that you can consider your treat on your 1600-calorie day:

2 pieces of whole-wheat bread or Ezekiel bread	180 calories
1 egg	90 calories
⅓ cup 2% milk	30 calories
dash of cinnamon	
½ tbsp of butter	60 calories
2 tbsp syrup	100 calories
½ piece or ½ cup of fruit	50 calories
Total	**510 calories**

> **Jim's French Toast**
>
> Directions:
> 1. Beat together egg, milk, and cinnamon.
> 2. Spray a griddle with nonstick cooking spray and turn stove to medium-high flame.
> 3. Dunk each slice of bread in egg mixture, soaking both sides. Place in pan, and cook on both sides until golden.
> 4. Top with butter and syrup.

Lunch

Many of my most successful Petites eat out for lunch almost every day. It's simply a part of their lives, whether they are eating out at work or socially with their friends and/or children. Personally, I eat out for lunch at least four or five times a week. Lunch will only vary by 100 calories. On you 1100-calorie days, it is 300 calories; on the 1600-calorie days, it only goes up by 100 to 400 calories. Here are some options.

Have a large salad. I have said this for years to Petites, but a salad is the perfect option for lunch, as it is easy to make, low in calories, and great for afternoon energy levels, since it's so easy to digest. And you can eat a lot. While I don't want to say that all vegetables are "free" calories, I do want you to know that you can eat a very large salad, as in six to eight cups of salad, for lunch and be perfectly on plan. Ideally, each salad, especially when eating in a restaurant, will include many different types of vegetables—peppers, broccoli, mushrooms, string beans, sprouts, etc. Determine the portion size of protein depending on the salad dressing you choose.

1 cup green raw peppers	30 calories
1 cup raw broccoli	31 calories
1 cup raw white mushrooms	15 calories
1 cup green string beans	34 calories
1 cup alfalfa sprouts	8 calories
1 cup cucumbers with peel	16 calories
1 cup cauliflower	25 calories
1 cup radishes, sliced	19 calories
1 cup cherry tomatoes	27 calories
1 oz boneless, skinless chicken	35 calories
1 oz Atlantic salmon	51 calories
1 oz pork tenderloin	40 calories
1 oz beef tenderloin	59 calories
1 oz tuna steak	30 calories
1 oz flank steak	44 calories
1 oz 90/10 ground beef	60 calories
1 oz 80/20 ground beef	77 calories
1 oz turkey breast	29.5 calories
1 oz firm tofu	22 calories

As you can see, you can eat far more boneless, skinless chicken, turkey breast, tuna, or tofu than you can of the other lean proteins. I give you this data, as I always want you to understand why I am recommending certain foods over others. I want you to have enough volume of food to satisfy you *and* give you the chance to enjoy other proteins like red meat when you have the desire to eat them.

Pay attention to salad dressings. It's really very easy if you simply ask for olive oil and either traditional vinegar (most restaurants serve red wine vinegar) or, ideally, balsamic vinegar. Ask for a separate bowl, or a coffee cup works very well. Pour one teaspoon of oil (as I'm sure there is a teaspoon on the table) into the cup and add as much balsamic vinegar as you like. Then add salt and pepper, but be careful with the salt. If you carry it, I love adding lemon pepper seasoning to dressing. You may also opt for balsamic vinegar only and add 1 ounce of blue, feta, or goat cheese. I love how they taste in salads and opt for them much more often than oil. I find I get more taste for my calories, and cheese contains protein, which the oil does not. Petite clients always tell me they opt for the cheese, as they get far more flavor per calorie than they get from the oil.

1 oz blue cheese	100 calories
1 oz feta cheese	75 calories
1 oz soft goat cheese	76 calories
1 oz Gorgonzola cheese	100 calories
1 oz cheddar cheese	114 calories

Another option for lunch is a turkey or chicken sandwich. Take two pieces of whole-wheat or Ezekiel bread or a whole-wheat wrap and add approximately four to six ounces of turkey or grilled chicken. At a major big-box grocery store, they sell pre-cooked strips of boneless, skinless chicken that I frequently place in a sandwich. Add to that as much lettuce, tomato, cucumber, or sprouts as you like (remember how low vegetables are in calories). Really load it up, as I want to keep you full. Then, finish it off with Dijon or another mustard (approximately 10 calories per teaspoon).

In most instances, the sandwich will chew up, literally, your 300–400 calories. That is why I want you to load the veggies on top. They are packed with fiber, water, vitamins, and nutrients that will give you great energy for the afternoon.

If you opt for an "open-face" sandwich, then you may have either:

- 2–3 oz more protein

- 1 piece of thinly sliced cheese

- 2 tsp mayonnaise (the real kind; you could have even more of a reduced-calorie version)

- 1 piece or cup of fruit on the side

Eggs are also a good choice for lunch. Try an omelet made with egg whites or with one whole egg and three whites. I frequently eat this for lunch, as I find it really fills me up. I order one egg and three whites to be cooked with a nonstick spray and have them add many different vegetables like spinach, broccoli, tomatoes (which really is a fruit), and sometimes even some feta cheese (1 ounce). With that, I generally eat half a cup of 1 or 2 percent cottage cheese, which is 160 to 180 calories per cup. It's a lot of tasty, low-fat protein and I sometimes just have to have something hot at lunch, especially when it's cold outside.

When eating lunch out (or in, for that matter), I *really* want you to avoid anything with mayonnaise, and that includes all tuna, chicken, and egg salad. Mayo is a lethal member of the Addies family. I've had struggling Petites tell me for years that they ate "light" and had a tuna fish sandwich. I almost needed oxygen. But I really don't blame them, as they were raised to believe that salads like these were diet foods. Sorry, but they were misinformed. Again, mayo is a highly caloric member of the Addies group and needs to be used very sparingly. If you can find a lower-calorie mayo or spread and use it in a portion-controlled manner, then that is fine. I have found that these are hard to find in the stores these days, so that is why I didn't include that option in the first place.

Dinner

For dinner, you can eat four to six ounces of protein (approximately 120 to 300 calories). Choose your portion and calorie count from the previous charts. To this, you can add three to five cups of vegetables chosen from the chart below.

1 cup green raw peppers	30 calories
1 cup raw broccoli	31 calories
1 cup raw white mushrooms	15 calories
1 cup green string beans	34 calories
1 cup cucumbers with peel	16 calories
1 cup cauliflower	25 calories
1 cup radishes, sliced	19 calories
1 cup cherry tomatoes	27 calories
1 medium sweet potato	100 calories

I want you to avoid rice in restaurants (with the exception of sushi, which I will explain later in this chapter), as it is always prepared with a lot of Addies like oil, butter, margarine, or other fat and that makes it very high in calories.

Let me break down what I consider to be the five components of dinner:

1. Bread. Note that this is *not* dipped in Addies. It's just plain old bread, hopefully whole-wheat or whole-grain, and also not Italian focaccia bread, which is "white" *and* loaded in oil, the king of Addies.

2. Appetizer. Make sure this is truly the size of an appetizer, not an entrée, and is absolutely not fried, filled with cream, or made in a phyllo-type dough.

3. Main course. An appropriate-size combination of lean protein, veggies, the right fats, and a "slow" carb.

4. Dessert. This is sorbet, not double-chocolate mocha cream-stuffed pie with crème fraîche.

5. Wine. Maximum 10 ounces—that means two 5-ounce glasses.

Here is how your restaurant dinner will affect your weight-loss plan. Be honest. Which of these sounds like you?

1 of the 5 components = a weight-loss day. Note that that can be the entrée with vegetables, fat, and the right "slow-release" carb.

2 of the 5 components = a weight-maintenance day. Note that if it's only one glass of wine instead of two, then it would fall into the weight-loss-day category.

3 of the 5 components = a slight overage of calories that can easily be burned off the next day by extra-careful calorie-counting.

4 of the 5 components = a larger overage of calories that will require three to five days of even more rigid calorie-counting plus potential added exercise.

5 of the 5 components = This alone may be the reason why you continue to gain weight.

Once again, I can just hear you saying: "Jim Karas just won't let me eat anything! He is spoiling all my fun." That's not true. My goal here is to help you and teach you to undo many of the not-so-great habits you have befriended in the past. Yes, I want you to have fun, but I also want you to succeed at this quest. Living "lean" is really *fun.* Just wait until you taste it. Trust me; it's amazing.

Eating Out Intelligently

Part of my goal in this chapter on eating out is to help you recalibrate your belief system and your vision of eating out. I can help you make it a great experience without suffering undue caloric damage. Once you get into this new "habit," you will be surprised at how easy it is to embrace. Since dinner is the most frequent meal eaten out in a restaurant, I want to tell you explicitly what to order in the most popular types of restaurants.

Steak houses

I *love* steak houses. Most Petites are shocked to hear me say that, if I had my way, you would eat every meal outside of your home in a steak house. Why? Because you don't have to play the "Avoid the Addies" game, as most food prepared in a steak house can be prepared "clean." When I use the word "clean," I mean prepared with little or no Addies. It's just great-quality, great-tasting food in its most natural state, with wonderful spices to enhance, not overwhelm, the taste. Your dinner at a steak house should include:

shrimp cocktail, 2 oz (about 4 small tails)	56 calories
4-oz filet or 5 oz of salmon	200 calories
8 large asparagus spears, 2 cups	91 calories
½ baked sweet potato, medium size (5" long by 2" wide)	50 calories
4 oz red wine	100 calories
Total	**497 calories**

This is *perfect* for your 1600-calorie-day dinner.

Petite busters: Portions. Steak houses are known for huge portions, so have your eyes finely tuned to the size of each dish that is coming to the table.

Mexican Restaurants

Mexican restaurants can be a great choice, if you avoid some obvious pitfalls. Here is what I want you to order and I will follow that with what I want you to avoid. Your dinner at a Mexican restaurant should include:

Chicken or shrimp fajitas (4 oz boneless, skinless chicken or shrimp)	149 calories
1 cup of chopped onions	64 calories
2 cups of green peppers	60 calories
1 corn tortilla	70 calories
1 tbsp olive oil	120 calories
10 tbsp salsa	40 calories (yes, that's 10 full tablespoons!)
Total	**484 calories**

This is *perfect* for your 1600-calorie-day dinner. And please, add lots of spices—cayenne pepper, red pepper chili flakes, or anything else spicy that you love.

Petite busters: Guacamole and the chips on the table. While avocado contains the "good" fat, it is a platinum member of the Addies and a little goes a long way. The chips on the table are deep-fried and packed with calories. Also, the rice and beans, while excellent if homemade with the right whole-grain or brown rice, are prepared with a tremendous amount of fat in restaurants and, therefore, are to be avoided.

Italian Restaurants

You probably already know that Italian restaurants are the most popular restaurants in the United States. This is good for the Italian restaurant owners and bad for your daily caloric intake, especially

if you are a Petite. Italian food is *very* difficult to manage in a restaurant. Here is your best bet:

4 oz of boneless, skinless chicken or fish	130–150 calories
1 tbsp of olive oil for preparation of meat or fish	120 calories
2 cups of grilled asparagus	54 calories
1 tsp of olive oil for preparation of asparagus	40 calories
1 5-oz glass of red wine	125 calories
Total	**489 calories**

This is *perfect* for your 1600-calorie-day dinner.

Petite busters: I need to take these one at a time since they
each present their own issue when it comes to Petites eating in
Italian restaurants.

- Bread. Most big, thick, Italian restaurant bread is a deal-breaker
  when it comes to a low-calorie meal. Similar to liquid calories
  (which I will address in chapter 7), if Americans would give up
  restaurant bread, our obesity epidemic would quickly flame
  out—at least somewhat. Most bread, especially the bread in
  Italian restaurants, is a caloric killer and, as I mentioned before,
  all white bread is a "quick empty" item.

- Olive oil. Back in the late 1980s, dipping your bread in olive oil
  became popular. That's a real disaster, as olive oil possesses
  more calories than butter (surprised?) and you just heard my
  opinion on bread. Everyone also assumed that, since olive oil
  is considered "healthy," you can eat as much of it as you want.
  I introduced you to my saying "Shine and glimmer won't make
  you slimmer" and the shine on your food in an Italian restaurant
  indicates just one thing—oil. If you find an Italian restaurant that

I had a well-known writer in New York City as a client. She was truly very good about her choices, portions, snacking, etc. She had only one major flaw; all her vegetables were prepared in oil, whether she was eating out or at home. Look, veggies are a terrific choice for many reasons, one of them being the fact that they are so high in water content. But when you cook veggies in oil, much of the wonderful water flies out and the unnecessary oil sucks itself in. That turns fifty calories of steamed spinach into 290 calories of spinach sautéed in olive oil. How did I arrive at that number? Olive oil (and all oil, for that matter) is 120 calories a tablespoon and 100 percent fat. Take two tablespoons in a saucepan, sauté the spinach, and presto, you just added 240 calories to the fifty-calorie spinach, for a total of 290 calories.

will prepare your food the way you want it, I say great. Go there whenever you get a craving for it. But in general, just know that Italian restaurants are going to pose a potential problem when it comes to the calories you plan to consume.

- Pasta. This one has to be avoided when eating out. It is all covered with Addies and the pasta alone is approximately 225 calories a cup. If eaten at home, without adding fat to the noodles, you should be fine. But in a restaurant, there is no way they will serve it to you without a great deal of added fat. Two tablespoons alone will make that one cup of pasta equal 465 calories. That's all you will get for your entire dinner—no fruits or vegetables, just simple carbs and fat. Not my recommendation for dinner.

Chinese Restaurants

Like Italian restaurants, Chinese eateries present a challenge. Not only is most of the food fried, but it is also frequently prepared in a lot of high-calorie sauce. Here is what I recommend:

1 cup of beef and broccoli	225 calories
½ cup of white rice (they virtually never have brown)	120 calories
2 pork or chicken pot stickers	150 calories
Total	**495 calories**

This is *perfect* for your 1600-calorie-day dinner.

Petite busters: Anything fried, like egg rolls and the majority of the chicken in many chicken dishes. Kung Pao chicken, the most popular dish eaten in Chinese restaurants, is sometimes as high as 1700 calories per container. Also, the brown sauce is made with cornstarch and other high-calorie Addies.

> ***Kryptonite was to Superman what variety is to Petites' desire to lose weight.*** *The variety makes you "weak" when you need to stay "strong." There are volumes of research that prove that the more variety presented, the more you will eat. In a Chinese restaurant, it is common to order a bunch of different dishes at the table and then to sample. That is not what I urge you to do as a Petite, because your dish must be carefully selected and prepared and you don't want to succumb to the "variety" issue.*

Thai Restaurants

Like Chinese restaurants, Thai restaurants limit your choices. But I find that you have more options in a Thai restaurant. Here is what I want you to order:

4 oz of chicken satay	120 calories
4 oz of shrimp	120 calories
OR	
4 oz of beef	200 calories
4 cups of steamed vegetables	120 calories
½ cup of white rice	120 calories
Total	**440 calories with beef; 480 calories with chicken and shrimp**

This is *perfect* for your 1600-calorie-day dinner.

Petite busters: Pad Thai, the noodle dish made with peanuts, is packed with calories, possibly as high as 1600 for one container. Anything made with coconut milk is also extremely high in calories and dangerous, saturated fat. The chicken satay is a great appetizer, but you have to skip the peanut sauce. The chicken alone has great flavor.

Greek Restaurants

Ah, now we are talking about my people. I am Greek and was raised in a household that served a lot of Greek food. The difference between the food served in Greece and the American version of it is unbelievable. Here is what I want you to order in a Greek restaurant:

Greek salad with 3–4 cups of vegetables	90 calories
½ oz of feta cheese	40 calories

½ tbsp of olive oil and 4 tbsp of vinegar	76 calories
4-oz chicken kebab	120 calories
OR	
4-oz beef kebab	200 calories
½ Greek roasted potato	60 calories
½ tbsp olive oil on the potato	60 calories
Total	**526 calories with beef;** **446 calories with chicken**

Again, a great dinner on your 1600-calorie day and also not bad if you cut a little of the oil for a 1100-calorie day.

Petite busters: Anything cooked in phyllo dough. I remember my grandmother making these cheese triangles that taste amazing. She would roll out the dough, then, with an industrial paintbrush, slather the butter on before rolling it up in the cheese. Also, like Italian food, anything made in a pan and anything with béchamel sauce, which is *über*caloric. Also, please pull the skin off the chicken, or any animal protein for that matter. Skin is a very toxic food that is not only loaded with fat, but all the wrong fat. Please always remove it; sometimes that is necessary in a Greek restaurant.

Sushi Restaurants

I treat sushi restaurants as a separate category, as I strongly recommend them for the combination of protein, carbs, and fat. Here is an ideal meal for you at dinner:

tuna roll (approximately 6 pieces)	180 calories
cucumber roll (approximately 6 pieces)	135 calories
avocado roll (approximately 6 pieces)	140 calories
Total	**455 calories**

That's eighteen pieces of sushi. It's a lot of food. And if you like, you can substitute one of the rolls for sashimi, which is simply the raw fish without the rice or seaweed. I know the rice is white, but I find that, in a restaurant, most brown rice is prepared with butter anyway, which pumps the calories up. Also, since the white rice is eaten with the protein and seaweed, the "quick empty" nature of the white carb slows down. You should also know that the seaweed is *packed* with vitamins and nutrients. It's an amazing anti-aging, anti-inflammatory food. I also really like the wasabi, as it also is packed with vitamins and nutrients and it tips satiety mechanisms, as do all spices. That is why sushi is generally a win-win choice.

Petite busters: The soy sauce, even if it is of the low-sodium variety. Regular soy sauce has approximately 1005 mg of sodium per tablespoon. The low-sodium variety is 600 mg. FYI, you should not consume more than 1500 mg of sodium a day. That is why you have to be careful with the use of soy sauce. If you mix a little in with your wasabi, you will find that just a dash goes a long way. The other Petite buster is anything labeled "spicy," as that generally means that it was prepared with mayonnaise, and we already talked about the danger of that when it comes to calories. I shouldn't have to say it, but tempura and all the fried items at a sushi restaurant are also off-limits. Not only is fried food in general high in calories, but it frequently is also cooked in the "wrong" oils that are full of saturated fats and also inflame the body. Remember how the leaves falling into a pool can clog up the baby pool more than the big Olympic pool? Well, fried food isn't just leaves falling into your baby pool. It's the whole tree!

I'm sure you see the themes that prevail with all my recommendations. Clearly, all portions must be on the smaller side. Add to that the case study from the New York University dietitians regarding the calorie and fat counts in most restaurants, and you have to agree. Frequently, when it comes to weight loss, I urge people to look to the past, when the average American was far lighter than we are now. I remember eating out as a little boy and frequently ordering "The Petite" filet. It was smaller than the big filet, which I could never finish. I still order "The Petite" filet to this day. I hope you now realize that you should as well.

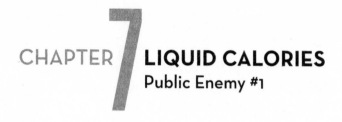

CHAPTER 7 LIQUID CALORIES
Public Enemy #1

A 2007 study reported in *Obesity* magazine showed that the average American is consuming 21 percent of their daily caloric intake in liquids.[1] Did you know that the average teenager is consuming between 500 and 1000 calories in liquid each and every day? That's a disaster for weight loss and is going to impact our teens negatively when they end up as obese, disease-ridden adults.

Studies by the Bloomberg School project that 75 percent of American adults will be overweight or obese by 2015 and they link liquid calories directly to the epidemic.[2] How's that for pointing the finger *directly* at liquid calories?

Petites, liquid calories are *killing* your desire to lose weight. This is true for almost all people, but even *more true* for you, because those extra liquid calories are *not* causing you to eat less. By that, I mean that neither your brain nor your body says: "I just drank a 200-calorie glass of juice, so I should eat less." Liquid calories are evil members of the Addies category and you know my feeling about them.

Here are two big reasons to avoid almost all liquid calories:

• Liquid calories do *not* tip satiety mechanisms.

• Liquid calories add up *very* quickly.

Numerous research studies have shown that calories consumed as liquid don't register a feeling of fullness (satiety) the way solid calories do. Translation: Wake up and drink orange juice (something you should *never* do) and your body says, "Where's the food?" Get up and eat an orange and your body says, "Thanks for the food."

Dr. Richard Mattes of Purdue University is at the forefront of this issue. He has conducted experiments using the solid form of food versus the liquid form of food with the exact same amount of calories and the same percentage of protein, carbohydrates, and fat. He and his team conclusively show that liquid calorie consumption does not lead to a feeling of fullness the way solid food does. In lay terms, you don't eat *or* drink; you eat *and* drink. And the calories you consume in liquid form do not have an impact on the amount of solids you chow down.

This is so important that I am going to reiterate it: When you eat a solid food, your body registers a certain feeling of fullness. When you consume the exact same food in liquid form (think eating watermelon versus drinking watermelon juice), your body does *not* register a feeling of fullness.

It is interesting to note that our American obesity epidemic coincided with both an increase in the size of servings of liquid calories (Big Gulp, anyone?) and the frequency with which we consume liquid calories (Starbucks all day, every day).[3] Are you one of these consumers? What does that tell you about your present body weight?

I will go so far as to say that if Petites would cease consuming liquid calories, they would immediately lose some weight. Possibly not *all* the weight they desire to lose, but they would make a significant dent.

Avoiding Liquid Calories

Almost every liquid calorie out there presents a danger, so let's take them one at time.

Water Bearing Calories

This is my fifth book, and never once in the past did I have to mention "water" when I talked about the evil of liquid calories. Unfortunately, there are a tremendous number of so-called "water" products that contain calories, and not just a few; some of them contain a *lot* of calories. You need to read labels before you just grab a water from a cooler. It's a shame you have to do that, but clearly someone is buying these waters or the stores wouldn't stock them.

Sports Drinks

Sports drinks are generally between eight and ten calories an ounce. They are a true marketing sham, as you do *not* need to replace electrolytes, etc. when exercising. Unless you are in the fifth set at Wimbledon against one of the Williams sisters—if you should be so lucky (or unlucky, as those girls are really something on the court!)—you should not be drinking them. FYI, nor should your children. Act as if they don't exist! It's another example of a food or beverage company telling us we need something that our ancestors didn't need in the past. I don't recall cowgirls drinking Gatorade out on the range, do you?

Soda

Soda is approximately twelve calories an ounce. According to the American Beverage Association, the average American drinks nearly fifty-four gallons of soft drinks each year. That, for the record, is the equivalent of almost twelve extra pounds of weight (probably *all* fat) each and every year. Another research study indicates that drinking just one soda a day increases your chances of obesity by 27 percent.[4] That's not a typo; just one soda a day increases your risk of obesity by 27 percent.

I am always shocked when I am on a plane, or at a party, or just people-watching and observe the staggering amount of soda people consume. I know women in their forties and fifties who drink over 100 ounces of real soda a day. Given that one sixty-four-ounce bottle of soda equals 960 calories, it's the equivalent of 100 pounds of fat, consumed by liquid—a year. Wow! Years ago, we had the wife of a major Chicago CEO as a client. She was a struggling, overweight Petite who was once a knockout. She became virtually unrecognizable as a result of her love affair with Pepsi, which she had no intention of breaking. Her flawed belief system led her to *believe* that Pepsi was not an issue. We finally had to just throw in the towel, which, FYI, is what her husband did a few years later. (She and Pepsi were recently seen vacationing together in Barbados.)

By now, you must be asking yourself: "What about diet soda?" Well, that's also not a great choice, as Lyn M. Steffen, Associate Professor of Epidemiology at the University of Minnesota found that the risk of metabolic syndrome—defined as the "triple threat" of high blood pressure, high blood sugar, and high cholesterol—increased by 34 percent in those who consumed just one diet soda each day compared to those who didn't drink any.

In another bit of similar researcher, Sharon P. Fowler, MPH, and colleagues at the University of Texas Health Science Center

> **I confess that I am a former diet soda-holic.** I used
> to pound at least 100 ounces of diet soda a day. It was a
> habit and I was hooked for many years. Moreover, I be-
> lieved that it wasn't hurting me. It wasn't until I stopped,
> cold turkey, that I realized how horrible it was making me
> feel. I was living on the caffeine highway most of the day
> with chronic ups and downs. Plus, my dentist looked at
> my teeth at my regular cleaning and exclaimed: "What
> have you been doing differently? They look great and I
> have less than half the usual work to do to get them back
> in shape." The only change I had made was cutting out
> diet soda.

studied 1500 people between the ages of twenty-five and fifty-four and found that drinking real soda (not diet) contributes to weight gain.[5] But, they also found that for each can of *diet* soda consumed, the risk of obesity went up by 41 percent.

The question remains: Is it something in the soda or it is more about the behaviors of those who choose to drink soda?

There is a body of research that points to the fact that the artificial sweeteners in diet soda may be playing with our cravings for sweets. Professors Terry Davidson and Susan Swithers from Purdue University found that rats that were fed artificial sweeteners "consistently ate more than the group fed high-calorie sweeteners."[6]

There is also a theory that, by consuming diet soda, we feel entitled to "treat" ourselves with other foods. You will hear a similar argument in chapter 8 when we talk about the damaging effects of cardiovascular exercise. I guess we can safely say that anyone drinking diet soda should:

1. Examine why they are drinking it, as they shouldn't be, especially if you are a Petite.

2. Look at what they could be drinking instead.

3. Determine if choosing diet soda is resulting in more sweet calories consumed in other areas.

Juice

Juice, in my opinion, is the worst possible liquid calorie you can consume. If you can believe it, juice is fifteen calories an ounce. That's 25 percent *more* calories than soda and almost twice the calories of sports drinks. People think that juice is "healthy." Almost every commercial juice is pasteurized to extend its shelf life and is generally chemically engineered to taste fresh. The pasteurization process heats up the juice and kills many of the valuable nutrients and vitamins. In addition, most fruit juices are only 10 percent juice; the rest is sugar. Eliminate juice. Ditto for your children or any children that you come across, for that matter, who have it in their little hands. Did you know that a tiny juice box with a straw possesses ninety calories? Take it away and replace it with water—not calorie water, but just water-water. That's what our kids need.

And just to finish this point, I don't even want you juicing at home. Eat the whole fruit. Not only will it tip satiety, it will also save you calories, as an average medium-size orange possesses sixty calories while an eight-ounce glass of orange juice has 120 calories. That's a 100 percent increase and your body doesn't even know it! Don't do it.

Calorie-Laden Coffee and Tea

Later in this chapter, you will learn that I am pro coffee and tea. For the record, that's plain coffee and tea, with nothing added but maybe a little sugar or a very small amount of artificial sweetener. But milkshakes masquerading as coffee or tea are not an approved beverage for Petites or anyone else for that matter. I have to say that, for Petites, even cream in coffee can be an issue if you are putting a lot of it into each cup and/or drinking a lot of coffee throughout the day. Be careful. Cream, even half-and-half (thirty-nine calories an ounce, and you may easily be using three ounces in each cup, which is 117 calories!) clearly falls in the Addies category and just adds up quickly.

Mixed Drinks—Especially Margaritas

In the next few pages, I am going to talk about alcohol, specifically wine. But this is about good old mixed drinks—gin and tonic, vodka and cranberry juice, margaritas, and cosmopolitans. These translate to *big* numbers when it comes to calories.

Mixed drinks are so calorically potent because you have to add the calories of the hard liquor—generally between 60 to 150 calories an ounce, depending on the proof—to the mixer, easily twelve to fifteen calories an ounce. Very quickly, your little "drink" adds up to hundreds of calories. Those big, frozen, albeit yummy, margaritas can add up to 500 calories each. That could be close to half your daily caloric intake. Think before you drink. No, better yet, think before you even order anything to drink that isn't water, or unsweetened tea or coffee. Say to yourself: "Do I really want to drink this, or am I just succumbing to peer pressure? Everyone else is drinking something. What should I do?" The answer to that last question is to decide what you really want, plug it into your daily caloric intake, and enjoy. I'm not a big fan of the old recommendation to drink a wine spritzer. To me, and to many Petites, that's like drinking Kool-Aid, because you can drink it so quickly and then want more.

Energy Drinks

Oy, the energy drinks and weight! Ladies, these drinks are lethal. They are packed with sugar and caffeine and cause all sorts of negative responses in the body. Once you "juice up" on them, your very smart brain says, "Wow, what's going on? You're on fire. We need to calm you down." Then it goes about doing so by releasing hormones and enabling you to slow down and not be so chemically "pumped." That will lead to a sugar *and* a caffeine crash and you will feel worse than you did before the drink.

Besides, these drinks, like the others I mentioned earlier, are calorie-packed. Petites just don't have that margin for error in their daily caloric intake. Don't drink them, buy them, or have them around the house, as *no one* needs to be drinking them! And, just like diet soda, I would be very leery of sugar-free energy drinks, as the same brain response may occur.

Drinks That Can Help You

I've spent the first part of this chapter telling you what *not* to drink. Now, it's time to get to what you can have.

Water

First and foremost is water. I know this must sound boring, but it's essential to your success. Look, this is *not* a new bit of advice, but so many Petites I know don't drink enough water. Plus, there is quite a bit of controversy as to how much water you should drink and what other liquids count toward your water balance. Let's examine the issues.

To determine how much water you should be drinking, I want you to get up tomorrow morning and weigh yourself. Then, I want you to drink half your body weight in water and, the very next morning, weigh yourself again. If the scale has gone down, then that indicates that you were holding on to water. The amount the scale has gone down indicates the amount of water you were holding, since you weren't drinking enough. Remember, I want to eradicate all water bloat, as that is part of what is keeping the scale up.

You see, the very smart human body holds water and you bloat when it is dehydrated. It does that as it senses there is not a readily available source of water, causing the brain to instruct the body to hold on to all available reserves. You can see the puff in your hands and feet, around your eyes and midsection, possibly everywhere. That is why staying in proper water balance is so very important—and especially important for those of you with a shorter stature. What looks like a little bloat on a taller woman looks like a *lot* of bloat on you. It's just like body fat. You don't have as much height to distribute it across. Therefore, you have to be that much more vigilant about your water balance.

Attention all "frequent flyers." *Cabin pressure is terribly dehydrating to your body. If you are about to fly, start drinking water. The fact that you have to get up to go to the bathroom frequently is good, since you don't want to remain sitting the whole time.*

Ditto to those of you who consume sodium, either in the foods you are choosing or by salting your food. Now, in my eating plan you will be on a low-sodium regimen, as I want you to see immediate results when you de-bloat. After your twenty-one days, I want you to continue to be vigilant about both sodium and water consumption, as they go hand in hand.

Just remember, bloat equals dehydration and should be your signal to start pumping down water immediately. You want to manage thirst. The only time you should feel thirsty is at the same time you feel hunger—first thing in the morning. I never want you to feel thirsty, because, at that point, you are already dehydrated. Clear urine is also a good indicator that you are in proper water balance.

The human body is made up of 60 to 75 percent water, and the brain is made up of even more than that. You *must* drink it, as it:

- Fills you up. I know you have heard it before, but it does. You want a feeling of fullness and water will help you to accomplish that.

- Burns calories. Researchers in Berlin found that drinking one half-liter of water (approximately a pint) burns an additional twenty-five calories a day.[7] While that may not seem like much, it clearly is going to add up over time. And remember, for Petites, every extra calorie burned counts. Plus, other research shows that cold water burns even more calories, since the body has to work harder to warm it up. I recommend that people drink virtually everything (and by everything, I mean water, unsweetened tea and coffee, and everything else) on ice. Not only will the ice add to your water intake, but cool liquids cause your body to burn more calories warming them up.

- Keeps you from drinking other lethal liquid calories. Instead of reaching for something packed with calories, reach for the gold standard—water. Just make sure, as I told you earlier, that it's not "water bearing calories."

- Keeps you from eating other calories. It has been found that some misinterpret hunger for thirst. The next time you are feeling hungry, try drinking a big glass of water instead of eating. That's what my leanest Petites do all the time. And then they do it as a routine that helps to ward off the hunger in the first place.

Tea

Tea is the second most consumed liquid in the world. I think that's great. Tea is an amazingly potent liquid as it helps to:

- Promote weight loss. Tea contains certain extracts, called catechins, that appear to increase metabolism. In a ten-year Taiwanese study, drinking black, green, or oolong tea just a few times a week resulted in 20 percent less body fat than in those who consumed a placebo beverage.[8] Catechins happen to be antioxidants, which promote health and slow the aging process, in addition to having many other properties that are beneficial to the body (I will talk about them shortly).

- Keep the weight off. A Dutch study found that drinking green tea helped people keep the weight off. Those in the study who drank a placebo regained as much as 40 percent of their lost weight, whereas the tea drinkers kept theirs off.[9]

- Boost exercise performance. A research study in Japan found that endurance doubled when mice were given green-tea extract as opposed to a placebo.[10] That's extremely important, as exercise intensity is critically important for Petites. Remember:

Intensity Up = Metabolism Up

- Repair muscles. You are about to learn that the key to a rockin' metabolism is to build those long, lean, calorie-burning muscles. Well, tea helps to repair them faster, enabling you to work out harder the next time. That will translate directly into more calories burned, as the muscle "repair" process is what burns so many calories.

- Increase "satiety." Research conducted in Sweden at Lund University studied adding green tea to exactly the same breakfast. After consuming bread and sliced turkey (which is something I actually eat often for breakfast or lunch), one group drank water while the other drank green tea. The green tea group reported a significantly higher feeling of satiety and less desire to eat their favorite foods.[11] That's a big plus for green tea, which I drink all the time—as do my most successful Petites.

- Promote numerous health benefits, including anti-aging, because it contains antioxidants.

Antioxidants, by definition, are "molecules capable of inhibiting the oxidation of other molecules. Oxidation is a chemical reaction that produces free radicals. Free radicals can start chain reactions that damage cells."[12] What that basically means is that antioxidants stop the damage that occurs to our cells. You may be shocked, but you increase the amount of this damage by doing a number of things:

1. Eating processed carbs, fast food, and/or trans fats.

2. Drinking damaging liquids—juice, soda, energy drinks, etc.

3. Sleep deprivation—which annihilates many things, including your cells.

4. Stress—a true killer.

5. Pollution—air, water, you name it.

6. Too much exposure to the sun.

7. Excessive exercise. Surprised? Most people are, but, while some exercise is essential, too much exercise is deeply damaging to your cells and body in general. Your best buddy who is exercising for hours and hours each week is actually doing more damage than good to her body.

It's that chain reaction that will diminish health and promote aging. So the goal is to stop, or at the very least slow, that process. Antioxidants do just that. Fruits, vegetables, and whole grains, as well as drinks like tea and coffee, contain many of these beneficial substances.

I pound hot and cold tea from morning until afternoon. I drink every possible type of tea and actually frequently play what I call the Tea Game. If I am giving a speech or at a meeting and notice that there are five different tea choices, I then go about drinking one cup of each type of tea, since they all have slightly different beneficial properties. I urge you to drink at least forty ounces of tea a day. That will probably be five glasses of iced tea or six glasses of hot tea.

Coffee

Coffee can be another beneficial liquid. Now, I don't mind coffee. The only issue is how coffee is affecting your energy levels and your sleep. If you need a cup of coffee to get you going in the morning, not a problem. Just make sure that it is not a cup of coffee laden with calories. But if you are on the coffee highway all day, drinking cup after cup to stay alert and awake, your adrenals may be affected, as well as your sleep.

If you are having difficulty sleeping, then coffee may be the culprit. Even decaffeinated coffee still possesses enough caffeine to get in the way of a restful night's sleep, so consider that if you are tossing and turning or popping up in the middle of the night. Start by cutting your coffee consumption in half and see if that helps. If it doesn't, then eliminate it, even though you will probably suffer caffeine withdrawal for the first few days.

Also know that all coffee is not the same. Starbucks coffee can have almost twice the caffeine (which is why people are so addicted to it) than other brands of coffee you either purchase or make at home. I'm not a coffee drinker, but I do know that the Starbucks

Black Tie gives me the jitters. I don't get the same response from green tea, so clearly there is a difference in the caffeine levels.

Milk

Milk is another beverage that can play a supporting role in a successful weight-loss plan—if you are careful. I know I've slammed liquid calories, but I feel that low-fat milk is an exception, as it possesses two positive applications:

- As a post-exercise snack. According to *Medicine & Science in Sports & Exercise,* drinking milk after exercising helped women drop three and a half pounds of fat in twelve weeks, compared to those who drank sports drinks and *gained* weight. Again, they gained weight with sports drinks, but lost weight with milk. Milk possesses whey protein, which is exactly what you want to consume after exercising on my program. On some days, you will see low-fat milk as one of your snacks post-exercise or just when you need to ward off hunger.

- For breakfast, coupled with high-fiber cereal. I know you are generally pressed for time at breakfast. A perfect, easy alternative (how hard is it to pour milk and cereal into a bowl?) is a good, high-fiber cereal with low-fat milk. Please note that I keep saying low-fat milk, as whole milk is loaded with the wrong fat and too many calories. Fat-free or skim milk does not tip satiety mechanisms. Some fat is *good* and low-fat milk is the perfect example. I generally recommend 2% milk.

Wine

It may surprise you that wine is also on the list of approved beverages. Okay, there is a lot of controversy surrounding alcohol. One camp says that moderate drinking, as in one glass a day, is fine.

Another camp says that moderate drinking can sometimes lead to more frequent, damaging drinking, so don't start in the first place. Then, other camps say "no" for religious, genetic, or health reasons, including an increased risk of certain cancers. I fall into the first camp and urge you to consider drinking a glass of wine from time to time, as we know wine has benefits such as:

- Improved heart health

- Increased good cholesterol

- Slowed cognitive decline

But did you know that one glass of wine can boost your metabolism? S. Goya Wannamethee, Ph.D. and epidemiologist at the Royal Free and University College Medical School in London, states that "alcohol may increase metabolic rate."[13] It appears that alcohol encourages your body to burn extra calories for up to ninety minutes after you drink a glass. That's why some studies find that regular wine drinkers have less abdominal fat, smaller waists, and a lower body mass index than those who don't drink wine. Drinking wine with a meal may actually result in more calories being burned rather than stored as fat. That, clearly, is a plus for Petites, and many of my personal training clients in Chicago and New York do drink a glass of wine two to three times a week.

The question for you is whether you enjoy drinking a glass of wine. I'm not a Petite, but I do. That, however, is a personal choice. While I have included wine in some of the eating-out options in my plan, you clearly don't have to drink it. I encourage you to increase the portions of the approved food slightly to equal the approximately 100 calories you save by not drinking the wine. Notice I didn't say *drink* something instead. "Unapproved" liquid calories are still just that—unapproved.

One final note on wine. Please, always be a "two-fisted" drinker. By that I mean, drink two ounces of water for every ounce of wine. When the human body breaks down alcohol, it uses water. By starting out well hydrated, you get up looking and feeling fine. That "groggy" feeling after you consume alcohol is often dehydration. By drinking two ounces of water for every ounce of wine, you will:

- Feel better.

- Look better, as you will avoid dehydration and the water "bloat" that comes with it. Hit the water and you will really see the difference in how you look in the morning.

- Drink less. Honestly, especially as a Petite, your small stature will fill up faster and that's good.

These two ounces of water equal ten ounces, since you should only be drinking five ounces of wine. That is in addition to the water I recommended earlier in the chapter.

Petites, please realize that what you consume in liquids is as important as what you consume in solids. Go back to your balance of energy equation and understand that your "calories in" come from both of them. Just one 8-ounce glass of juice each day adds up to 96 calories a day, 35,040 calories a year, and ten extra pounds. OUCH! Substituting "liquid bearing calories" with water and tea will not only save you calories, it will lean you out and give you the visual that will keep you coming back for more. Here is your new mantra—the right liquids enable you to "blast the fat" and "beat the bloat."

CHAPTER 8 EXERCISE
A Petite's BFF

My exercise program is going to make you "tighter and lighter." And that's why, for the first time in your life, you are going to experience not only weight loss; you are also going to experience your first "recomposition."

Let me clarify. I have had countless Petites tell me, sometimes in tears:

- I really didn't tone up. I didn't look even remotely like the pictures I was promised.

- I looked pretty much the same, only a touch smaller. I've always been shaped like a pear. Then after losing a little weight, I basically just looked like a slightly smaller pear. And after all that time I spent on the treadmill!

- I still have jiggling skin. I don't want to wear sleeveless tops, even though I was promised that I could. I hate my thighs, so continue to avoid shorts. I don't really feel that much better about myself.

- I actually preferred how I looked heavier. I seemed more "out of proportion" as I lost weight, mostly from the top down. The weight I had to lose was in my lower half. Now I have smaller breasts and the same size legs. After just slight weight loss, my lower half looked even bigger. What's the point in losing weight if that's my end result?

Ladies, I couldn't agree with you more. Why follow a plan and end up unhappy? Clearly, you did not witness a "recomposition" of your body, probably because you made one of two errors in the past: either you didn't exercise, or you performed cardiovascular exercise.

I know I made this point earlier, but it warrants repeating. If you diet without exercise, you destroy your metabolism because you are losing almost as much muscle as fat—not that ugly, bulging muscle you see in all the wrong magazines, but rather the beautiful, long, elegant muscle that you see on certain women and wonder what their secret is. I have the secret. Just wait a moment longer.

The Dangers of Cardiovascular Exercise

The other mistake you may have made is to perform cardiovascular exercise. As the author of the *New York Times* bestseller *The Cardio-Free Diet*, I am here to tell you definitively that classic cardiovascular exercise is a complete and utter waste of time if your goal is weight loss and a "recomposition." I don't want to go into the complete argument, but suffice it to say that cardio kills, which was the original title to the book. (I wish we had kept it, as it truly represents my opinion.) Cardiovascular exercise can have deeply damaging effects.

First, it can destroy your joints. Just look at all the runners limping around and complaining about their backs, knees, etc. According to the *New York Times*, the #2 reason why baby boomers (approximately 78 million Americans) go to the doctor is for an exercise-related injury.[1] Consider these horrible statistics regarding marathoners:

- 25 percent of all people who begin to train for a marathon have to drop out due to injury.

- 19 percent of all those who run a marathon (I truly feel sorry for them for completing this deeply damaging event) suffer an injury.

If you work the math—which by now you know I love—you will see that, if 100 people attempt to run a marathon, twenty-five will quit because of injury and 19 percent of the remaining seventy-five (approximately fourteen) will also be injured. That means that, out of the original 100 people, thirty-nine will be injured—a 39 percent injury rate. And trust me, from my experience in this industry, I know that the number is even higher than that. That doesn't even take into account the damage that occurs over time, as the vast majority of marathon runners require hip or knee replacements at some point due to wear and tear on those joints. Clearly, this is not a smart option if your goal is to exercise for life in order to stay lean for life.

Moreover, excessive cardio decimates your immune system. Now, to be fair, twenty to thirty minutes of cardio can enhance your immune system, but anything over that leads you in the wrong direction. Why do you think so many marathon runners get sick after a race? A drop in immunity is the only logical explanation.

And what about posture? If I see one more person hunched over running or, better yet, hanging on a stair stepper, treadmill, or

> **The question of cardiovascular exercise** *goes back to the whole issue of belief systems. According to the Washington Post, over 100 million Americans embraced cardio in the "new fitness revolution" of the 1980s—which also happens to correlate with the time when our obesity epidemic skyrocketed. That's over thirty years ago. So we have thirty years of evidence that shows that cardio doesn't work for weight loss. Why, then, would anyone, especially a Petite, regularly hit the pavement, sign up for a spin class, or jockey for position in ZUMBA? I don't know. I guess we are back to the definition of insanity and a painfully flawed belief system.*

spin bike, I will explode. Why do they think that performing that activity makes them look good when it doesn't? Is your goal to have hunched-forward shoulders with a neck that juts out and a puffy stomach with matching thighs? I hope not—but that's what you get from all the mindless, posture-destroying cardio.

Posture is critically important to you as a Petite. You need every possible eighth of an inch so that you can optimize the height you have been given. That is why my exercise program specifically enhances your posture. When you follow my plan, you will perform two exercises for the back of your body for every one exercise for the front. That will result in great posture and you will love the way you look and feel. Right now, just take a look at yourself in a mirror as you pull your shoulders back and down. That's what you will look like all the time.

Cardiovascular exercise can also potentially damage your heart. A very recent study in Britain looked at the hearts of mar-

athon runners versus more sedentary men. What they found through magnetic resonance imaging was a great deal of damage called fibrosis in the hearts of the marathoners. Fibrosis is scarring within the heart muscle, which, if severe, can lead to thickening or stiffening of some portions of the heart. This can contribute to irregular heartbeat and, in some instances, heart failure. Researchers found that the more the men in the study ran, the more they showed evidence of scarring, or fibrosis.[2] Why then, would anyone of sound mind and body lace up a pair of running shoes to perform a marathon or any excessive amount of cardiovascular exercise? It just doesn't make any sense. And remember, your delicate, smaller stature gets hit that much harder by various behaviors and activities. For Petites, excessive cardio can lead to tragic outcomes.

Cardio also destroys muscle. No, I am *not* kidding. After twenty to thirty minutes of cardio, your body starts to chew up its precious muscle—and you know my opinion of anything that burns up muscle! Along with the muscle goes your metabolism and any desire to live in "The Land of the Lean." I go into far more detail in *The Cardio-Free Diet* about this critical issue, so take a look at it if you have the opportunity.

But wait! I want to be clear. There is one thing that cardiovascular exercise doesn't destroy—*your appetite*! Research has shown this for years. When *Time* magazine's August 17, 2009 cover story appeared with the title, "Does Exercise Make You Fat?" I never felt so vindicated. Yes. The research shows that cardiovascular exercise is a disaster when it comes to weight loss, as all it does is make you hungry. In fact, you quickly eat up the few calories you did manage to burn performing cardio—and then you eat lots more!

There is so much research to cite that we can't consider it all here, but let me give you just a tease. Danish researchers published a weight-loss study in 1989 that took a group of nonathletes and

trained them for eighteen months to run a marathon. Upon completing the training, the men had lost five pounds, but the women had lost nothing—zip, nada—although they had trained for eighteen months as well.[3] What does that say about cardio for weight loss? I think it says it doesn't work. In fact, there is other research that shows that cardio can lead to weight *gain*.

The *Time* article highlighted two behaviors that are directly attributable to two flawed beliefs:

- *"I exercised, so hey, I can eat!"* At Jim Karas Personal Training, we call this "playing for the tie." It doesn't work and most people continue to gain weight. And once you've injured yourself with all that cardio, which is all but inevitable, you will really start to pile on the pounds as you continue to eat with reckless abandon. I know many people who literally "treat" themselves with 800-calorie snacks (FYI, that's a classic cappuccino and a muffin) after burning 250 calories. It's easy to see that that's not going to lead to anything but weight gain when you plug it into the balance of energy equation!

- *"I exercised, so hey, I don't need to move around as much for the rest of the day! I can just sit around all day."* We already know the evil of sitting when it comes to your health and body weight. Also, remember my favorite research on the Seven Behaviors of Successful Weight Loss. People who successfully lost weight were active for ninety minutes each day. If you perform useless cardio for thirty minutes and burn next to no calories, then sit around for the rest of the day, you are truly destined to getting bigger and bigger.

And I want to chime in with one more point about cardio: you *do* get hungry. Where do you think the phrase "working up an

appetite" comes from? Cardiovascular exercise will never lead to weight loss. Go back to the weight-loss equation:

Calories In - Calories Out

Sure, you do burn a few calories performing cardio (and FYI, all the machines lie about the amount of calories you are burning, so don't believe them). But if you then overeat on the "calories in" part of the equation, you'll never get to a caloric deficit, which is what weight loss is all about. You actually have the perfect equation for a long-term caloric surplus—AKA, weight gain.

Exercise for Weight Loss

Okay, we agree, cardio is out, but, you absolutely *must* exercise or I wouldn't call it your BFF.

Let's go back to the beginning.

I stated that weight loss is 75 percent eating and 25 percent exercise. But, without the style of exercise prescribed in this chapter, your likelihood of success is minimal. No, I will go so far as to say that your likelihood of long-term weight loss is near zilch and there is no way you will experience a "recomposition" of your body.

When *The Cardio-Free Diet* came out in 2007, it shot to #2 on the *New York Times* bestseller list and caused a great deal of controversy. My biggest critics were doctors, who said, well, less than pleasant things about my theory. They said I was neglecting heart health. I have to laugh, as many of them were overweight, yet passionate about their belief that classic cardio is essential to weight loss and heart health. Talk about a flawed belief system! They attacked my theory on strength training, but didn't read the book or even perform the exercises in it that produce such astonishing results. They just kept repeating: "You have to perform cardio for heart health, you have to perform cardio for heart health …"

Here is a bit of research that drives my point home.

Researchers at the Department of Human Performance and Applied Exercise Science at West Virginia University examined the effects of a very-low-calorie diet (800 calories a day, and we know that's *low*). They broke seventeen women and three men up into two groups for a twelve-week study:

- Group 1 consumed the very-low-calorie diet and performed cardiovascular exercise four times a week for one hour by walking, biking, or stair-climbing.

- Group 2 consumed the same very-low-calorie diet and performed strength training three times a week, increasing from two sets of eight to fifteen repetitions of ten exercises (with only one minute of rest in between) to four sets of eight to twelve repetitions (remember this number) by the end of the study.[4]

By the end of the twelve-week period, oxygen consumption increased significantly but *equally* in both groups. That means that both groups got into better cardiovascular shape. That's what all my critics failed to realize. Progressive strength training three times a week provided the same cardiovascular benefits as the cardio performed four times a week for one hour. *Both groups experienced the same heart-health benefits.* How can you neglect this research and claim that I am "anti heart health" when the research totally agrees that strength training achieves the same heart-health benefits as cardio? And this is only one research study. There are dozens more out there.

Moreover, group 1, the cardio group, experienced a significant reduction in lean muscle tissue and in resting metabolic rate.

Remember:

Muscle Down = Metabolism Down

Therefore, cardio plus a very-low-calorie diet resulted in muscle loss. This is precisely what I believe to be the major problem with long-term weight loss—with or without cardio. Both strategies result in a reduction in your lean muscle tissue and therefore a reduction in your metabolism. Unless you are committed to eating very little for the rest of your life (which is not what I recommend), you are doomed to gain all the weight back and then some—and it's all going to be *fat*.

Moreover, without the strength training, you probably won't even like what your body looks like at your lower weight, as you won't have caused a "recomposition" to occur. Without a "recomposition," your body will most likely be sagging, puckering, and out of proportion—not what you set out to accomplish—because you didn't perform the results-producing exercise program in this book.

Remember from our earlier discussion of metabolism that when you *do* gain weight back after dieting, it will be all fat. You probably would have been better off never having lost the weight in the first place, as you now are at the same high weight with a decimated metabolism, just like turning your hair dryer or blender on *low*!

In the West Virginia study, group 2—the strength-training group—did *not* experience a decrease in lean muscle tissue or metabolism. This is very significant, given that the participants were only consuming 800 calories a day. On my plan, you are getting 1100–1600 calories a day. So this provides just one more example of the fact that you *can* go even as low as 800 calories and not affect your metabolism if you perform strength training. It's almost mind-boggling, but the researchers were quick to point out that the participants in group 2 progressed (increased both the weight and the reps) in their strength-training programs. Thus they kept challenging their muscles. They noted that other case studies did not show an increase in lean muscle tissue for those performing strength training while on a very-low-calorie diet. They indicated, however, that those participants did not continue to challenge their muscles and their bodies by increasing both the weights and the reps. They just did a routine (which is a four-letter word when it comes to strength training) and didn't increase the intensity as their bodies adapted to the exercise. Progression is essential, because:

Progressive Strength Training = Increased Lean Muscle Tissue

Increased Lean Muscle Tissue = Revved-Up Metabolism

Revved-Up Metabolism = Petites' Permanent Weight Loss

Now let's dive into your exercise program.

Interval Strength Training

Intervals are the key to optimizing many things, including heart health. What irritates me about many doctors, therapists, and personal trainers who challenge me on my cardio-free position is that they don't even attempt to perform the exercises I have outlined. If they did, they would realize that their heart rate really goes up when performing these programs and that exercising in intervals provides even more heart health than classic, steady-state, useless cardiovascular exercise. They ignore the research that shows that regular strength training, with one minute of rest between each set, provides just as much heart health as cardio.

Your interval-based strength-training program will also start with one minute of rest between each exercise. When you start to apply progression to this plan, you will perform these exercises

with only thirty seconds of rest between each set. By doing
you will derive even more heart health and even more post-ex
calorie burn.

Each exercise in this program requires approximately one minute to perform a ten-repetition set, followed by one minute of rest
as you prepare for the next exercise. That one minute of exercise
followed by one minute of rest constitutes the *interval,* as your
heart rate will go up and then decline when you are resting. It's a
bit like a classic roller coaster that goes up and down, up and down.

I am a big fan of heart-rate monitors. But traditional heart-rate
monitors require that you wear a chest strap, of which I have never
been a big fan. Many of my clients told me that they loved the
information they got from the heart-rate monitor, but found the
chest strap uncomfortable. Now, a new monitor has been created
that only requires that you touch the monitor to obtain your heart
rate. Go to www.JimKaras.com for details.

I have always been a fan of what Diane Sawyer calls "measur-
able results." Diane was very clear to me at our initial consultation
at her home that she needs to see quantifiable details as to how
her body is responding to the eating and exercise program that I
put her on. She wore the heart-rate monitor initially, but disliked
the chest strap, so I took her readings manually.

The reason a heart-rate monitor can be so beneficial is that it
shows you how your heart rate jumps up during exercise, then how
it responds during periods of rest. Thus, you can see very quickly
that you body starts to get into better shape. Your whole cardiovascular system improves, which is good news. The bad news is
that this then requires you to work harder to achieve the same
heart rate. I know you don't want to hear that you have to work
hard, but—come on—if this were easy, would anyone be overweight?
Yes, you have to work hard, but trust me: the amazing results are
so worth it that you will keep coming back for more.

And being a Petite does make exercise easier for you. Your compact stature makes you strong and coordinated. You will fly through this program and it will feel like dancing, which is something I really love and hope you do as well.

So what exactly is strength training? I find that most people are totally confused by the term, so let me break it down for you.

Strength Training 101

Strength training consists of three phases: working repetitions, fatigue, and failure. Yes, that's right: failure. Let me explain.

In the first phase of strength training, you will easily complete approximately the first five or six repetitions of your ten-rep set. You are in good form, it is not too hard, and you are moving at a pace that correlates approximately to a count of one one thousand, two one thousand, three one thousand on the concentric—when you are contracting or shortening the muscle—and the same on the eccentric—when you are lengthening the muscle and returning to the starting position. That is why each set in my program will take approximately one minute. Since it will take you three seconds to contract (shorten) the muscle and three seconds to lengthen the muscle, each rep will take you 6 seconds. Since you will perform ten repetitions of each exercise:

6 Seconds per Rep x 10 Repetitions = 60 Seconds or 1 Minute

Speed is a big issue when it comes to effective strength training. Many people I see go far too fast when performing their routines. As a result, they are just using momentum, not muscle—and they are also risking injury. The expression "slow and steady" applies perfectly to effective strength training.

You will also be working a full range of motion for each repetition, which means that you will be working through the full range of each muscle group. Full range of motion is the key to developing long, lean, sexy muscles and to improving your posture.

In phase 2—fatigue—you will start to really feel the muscle around the sixth, seventh, or eighth repetition. This may include some burn and possibly a desire to cheat, or use other muscle groups to help you out, or cut down on the full range of motion. Your muscles are clearly telling you: "Hey, this is getting *really* hard." This is good, as you are overloading the muscle (that's the key to strength training) and nearing the most critical part of the training.

In phase 3—failure—you hit momentary muscular failure and can no longer perform even one more repetition to continue the set. This is extremely important because, when it comes to strength training:

You Succeed When You Fail!

Failure is essential to strength training, as it sets into play two important responses by the body.

1. When you hit the essential "failure," you create tiny little tears in your muscle fibers. Don't think of a tear as a bad thing. On the contrary, breaking down and tearing muscle fiber is your goal, because then, over the next twenty-four to forty-eight hours, the muscle fiber will go about repairing itself.

2. As the muscle fiber repairs itself, your very smart brain says to your body: "Hey, the next time you perform that strength-training exercise, I want you to get better at it, or more proficient." It therefore tells your body, while repairing the muscle fibers, to slightly increase the amount of lean muscle tissue. This increase in lean muscle tissue will give you more strength *and* the increase in your metabolism you so desperately need and desire. It's a win-win situation.

Please reread what I just wrote expressed as an equation:

More Strength = More Lean Muscle Tissue

More Lean Muscle Tissue = Increased Metabolism

If your intensity and strength is staying the same or increasing, then your lean muscle tissue is staying the same or increasing. There is only one tissue you are losing—*fat*. That's great and is your goal on this plan. If your strength and intensity go down, that's an indication that you are losing muscle. Strength and muscle are best friends. They go up and down in tandem.

Now, to be perfectly clear, the vast majority of people that I see performing what they think is strength training never hit this critical failure phase because they use very light weights. Using very light weights is a *total* waste of time. You need to use a tension/weight that enables you to hit failure by the tenth repetition. Remember:

More Tension = More Results

When I talk about the "magic" of strength training, most women say to me: "Oh Jim, I already strength train." Then they proceed to tell me about a program they embraced in 1972 that urged them to use three-pound weights. They have never lifted more than three pounds and they call that strength training! Please understand, it's not.

Performing too many repetitions goes hand in hand with using very light weights. You must abandon the belief system that says light weights and many reps "tones" the muscle, while heavy weights and fewer reps "builds" the muscle. This is an old wives' tale and is totally untrue. You *want* to build muscle, because slightly increasing your lean muscle tissue and burning off all your body fat is what is going to create that "toned" look. I will go so far as to say that heavier weights/tension works magic on your body, regardless of your age, height, or weight. Jane Brody, a health writer for *The New York Times*, has written that "strength training gives women a tighter physique." That's the "recomposition" you're going to experience.

Other mistakes people make when they think they are doing strength training is to lift too quickly and to ignore form. Never, ever lift weight rapidly. You want to move slowly to "overload" the muscle effectively, which is what you accomplish when you hit the fatigue and failure phases. That "overload" requires what we call "time under tension." For each set, you will give your muscles sixty seconds or less to fail.

And remember to emphasize form. The key to effective strength training is to isolate the muscle that you are challenging. If your form is all over the place while you are watching TV (which you will *not* be doing while performing my exercise routine, as I would much rather have you listening to music), you are pretty much wasting your time and risking injury. I'm only asking you to exercise for thirty-one minutes, three times a week. Clearly, you can focus your attention for thirty-one minutes on this results-producing activity. And the appearance of those sexy muscles will keep you coming back for more.

By performing strength training my way, you will find that the time just flies by and you see results right away, especially if you are very new to strength training or now performing it the right way for the first time.

Remember that, as a Petite, you are generally more athletic than many taller women. You are known to be faster, more flexible, and more structurally aligned (the taller you are, the greater your risk of injury). Therefore, you can hit this exercise program hard, as intensity is so essential to seeing and feeling the results you desire.

Intensity is critically important, because we want to optimize not just the calories you burn during the exercise, but the calories you burn after the exercise. This after-burn—technically called EPOC, Excess Post-Exercise Oxygen Consumption—is the most important element of exercise. By performing just thirty-one minutes of my interval-based strength training, you may experience a thirty-eight-hour increase in your metabolism. No, that's not a typo. Thirty-eight hours *after* you have exercised, your metabolism will still be pumping at a rate higher than normal.

You may be wondering why. Why such a response? It is caused by something called "disruption." When you perform these exercises, you shock your system, confuse your muscles, cause a great deal of disruption, and subsequent muscle-tissue damage. Then, the "repair" process that I mentioned earlier comes into play, which requires a lot of calories and bumps up your metabolism. As a Petite, it is essential that your metabolism is always pumping. Remember, we want your motor on "high" all the time, just like your hair dryer and blender. You can't create the big caloric deficit that taller women can, therefore, your "calories out" have to be high. That's why your EPOC is so important. FYI, the EPOC of cardio is only a few hours—yet another reason why it's a complete and utter waste of time.

Gravity Straps

I specifically selected the Gravity Straps as the equipment for this program because it is perfect for Petites:

- It allows you to set the intensity. By changing your foot positioning, you can make the exercise more or less challenging or intense. Know that intensity is your best friend. You never really saw results in the past because you never really challenged yourself. This routine is a great challenge and Gravity Straps are the perfect tool to accomplish your "recomposition."

- You determine the range of motion. Given your smaller stature, I don't want you to feel confined to a program or piece of equipment that you have to try to fit into. You are in complete control of the range of motion that you need to build those long, lean, sexy muscles and stay motivated.

- It works the whole body, all the time. You want to stimulate as many muscles as possible. By using your body weight at all times, you fire up so many muscles that both the calorie burn during the exercise program *and* the after-burn are off the charts.

- You really challenge your core. Since you are standing at all times, you are forcing your core to work. The more you work it, the more you will love the new shape of your body. You want that tight, sexy, hourglass figure. The more you lean out your midsection, the more you will love the way you look.

- You very effectively work the back of your body. Posture is critical to a Petite. I call posture your "Weapon of Mass Retraction," because scapular retraction literally means pulling your shoulders back. This piece of equipment allows you to work the back of your body very effectively, which is the key to perfect posture and to stretching out and elongating the front of your body.

Because we spend our lives in our cars, at computers, and carrying purses, briefcases, luggage, groceries, and kids, we spend *too much time* hunched forward. We tighten up our chest and shoulder muscles and that brings our posture forward and down. That is not the goal. The goal is the complete opposite. You want your chest open, your shoulders back, and your head held high and in alignment. Improving your posture immediately leans out your abdominals, as you are standing up straighter and therefore lengthening those core muscles in the front. And every eighth of an inch makes a difference.

When you follow my exercise plan, you are working the two sides of your body individually. We call this "unilateral" training in the industry. We all have a dominant side. By using the individual handles of the Gravity Straps, your stronger arm cannot take over. You probably have one arm that is longer than the other and ditto for your legs. These exercises will keep you in perfect balance, and better balance leads to more strength.

More Strength = More Muscle

More Muscle = Increased Metabolism

And that all means one word that we *all* love to hear—***results!***

I also love this product because it travels well. Whether you travel for business, for pleasure, or for family, any piece of exercise equipment that is easy to transport will get more use. I've traveled with this for years and my most successful Petites know that exercise is not an option—and that includes when you are away from home. The Gravity Straps weigh next to nothing, so it's not a weight issue in your suitcase or carry-on when traveling. It's a "Petite" piece of equipment. It even comes with a carrying case, so it's perfect for all your needs.

With this piece of equipment, all you need is a door. And you can move it to different locations in your house as well. If you have to keep your eye on the kids or move to another part of your home for privacy or sunlight, you can just bring it along. You can even attach it to your back door when the sun is out. Sunlight is extremely important to your circadian rhythm (your sleep/wake cycle) and to your energy levels. Besides, it just feels good to exercise outside in the fresh air.

The Exercise Program

There are three components to this exercise program that are specifically designed for Petites:

Dynamic Warm-Up. In the past, many people wasted their time on a useless piece of cardiovascular equipment to warm up, pounding their joints and causing a horrible jarring motion throughout their bodies. They also generally started hunched over, so the first thing they told their minds and bodies was to round their shoulders forward and jut out their heads. That is exactly what you are *not* going to do with this plan. Right from the start, you are going to *prepare* your body for the exercise and immediately tell it: "We are going to pull everything back in a kind, gentle, and effective manner." In this way, once you move into the more intense portion of the program, your body is ready for the activity.

Core. For a Petite, the key to that sexy hourglass figure that feels great both in and out of clothes is your core. It should be proportionate and look exactly like a woman's figure should look. By reducing your whole core—front, back, *and* sides—you get that tight midsection that I'm sure you thought was out of your reach. We'll go through these core exercises right after the dynamic warm-up, as I really want you to use every available bit of energy to hit them hard and effectively. Clearly, your energy levels will be at their peak right after your warm-up, as your available fuel (glucose) is ready to give you power. By hitting your core early and hard, you will work the most important part of your program. You will be working your core throughout this program, however. These are just the exercises that are the most specific.

The Full-Body Strength-Training Program. These are the exercises that fire up your entire body. You will notice that, frequently, your whole body is working at once. In that way, you stimulate the maximum amount of muscle fiber (which is what you tear and then repair and regrow) in the minimum amount of time. Remember, exercise is stress. You want to minimize the stress, but derive the optimum benefits.

Many of the exercises that follow are familiar. You will be performing many variations on exercises you already know—squats, lunges, push-ups, back rows, and planks. But with the Gravity Straps, you can make them that much more effective and fun.

The "Petites" Exercise Plan

How to Attach the Gravity Straps

The Gravity Straps come with two individual straps. Each strap needs to be attached to the top of your door, and then you close the door securely. Have no fear, as the weighted back side of the Gravity Straps keeps it firmly in place. You may need to adjust the straps for some of the exercises and I will make notes when that will be necessary.

For all exercises, perform 10 repetitions, unless instructed otherwise, to the speed indicated.

Dynamic Warm-Up

1. Overhead V Squat

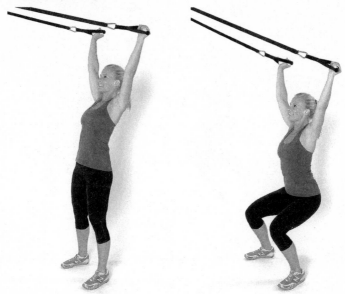

a. Start with your feet shoulder-width apart, shoulders back, and abs tucked.

b. With one strap in each hand, palms facing forward, place your arms over your head as if you are creating the letter V.

c. Make sure the tension is very taut when your arms are up.

d. Slowly start to lower down into a squat until your hamstrings, the backs of your legs, are parallel to the floor.

e. Remember that you are moving slowly to a three count, so it is one one thousand, two one thousand, three one thousand on the way down, pause for a beat, then the same speed as you return.

f. Inhale on the way down, exhale on the way up.

g. Make sure to pull in your abdominals at all times.

h. Tension should be in your back, shoulders, and core.

2. *Hip Extension to Y Shoulder Raise*

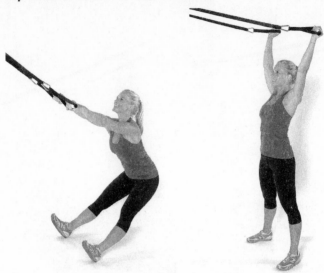

a. Start with your feet shoulder-width apart, shoulders back, and abs tucked.

b. With one strap in each hand, palms facing down, lean back, hinging at your hip.

c. Make sure that the tension is very taut when your arms are extended.

d. Slowly start to lift your body up, keeping the legs straight, which is very different from your first exercise, arms over your head as if you are creating the letter V.

e. In this instance, you are moving slightly faster than your first exercise. Perform a two count, so it is one one thousand, two one thousand, on the way up, no pause, then the same speed as you return.

f. Inhale on the way down, exhale on the way up.

g. Make sure to pull in your abdominals at all times.

h. Feel the stretch in your arms, back, glutes, and legs in the lowering phase, then feel the tension in those same muscles as you pull yourself up.

NOTE: As I mentioned in the earlier text, I just love exercises for Petites that lengthen then strengthen your muscles. Repeat that in your head as you are performing many of these exercises: "Lengthen then strengthen" to create that long, lean visual we all admire and aspire to possess.

Progression

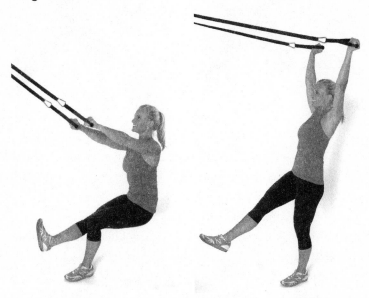

a. To begin, stand on the left leg with the left knee slightly bent, as pictured.
b. Extend the right leg with your heel digging into the floor.
c. Then, lift up, as you did when on both legs, but this time, only use the left leg as the right leg will lift up and extend straight out in front of you, as pictured.
d. Perform the first 5 reps on the right leg, then switch to the left.

This is a tough movement, so don't be surprised if you can only perform a few on each leg, then finish out the set on both legs.

3. *Lateral Squats*

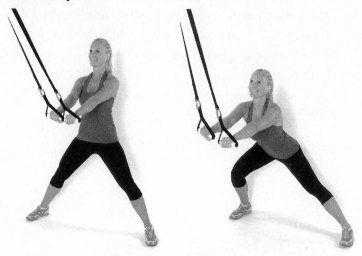

a. Start with your feet wide, toes slightly turned out, shoulders back, and abs tucked.

b. Extend your arms straight out in front of you with your hands in each individual strap, palms down.

c. Make sure that the tension is very taut when your arms are extended.

d. Slowly start to side lunge over to your right side, hold for one count, then move slowly over to the left side.

e. This exercise moves to a two count, so it is one one thousand, two one thousand on the way to the right, no pause, then the same speed as you shift to the left.

f. Inhale on the way to the right, exhale on the way to the left

g. Make sure to pull in your abdominals at all times and don't let your shoulders round forward. Fight to keep them back, as that is a big part of this movement.

h. Don't be surprised if you feel this in your back, arms, core, and legs. This movement is firing up a lot of muscles at the same time, but remember, that's your goal, as intensity sheds fat and inches.

Progression

a. Assume the exact same position, but hold both straps in one hand.

b. Start with the right hand, and perform 5 reps (one complete rep is going from the right to the left and back), then switch to the left hand for the remaining five.

You will find that you have to fight that much harder to maintain proper posture and positioning (say "proper, posture, positioning" really fast 10 times!).

You will also experience more challenge to your core, which will help to give you that hourglass figure.

4. Squat to Row

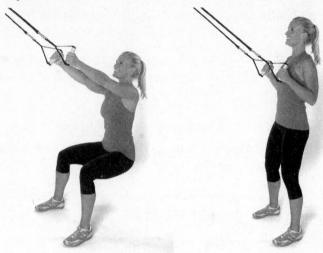

a. Start with your feet shoulder-width apart, shoulders back, and abs tucked.

b. Place your hands in the straps with palms facing each other and squat down until your glutes almost hit the floor, as pictured.

c. Make sure that the tension is very taut when your arms are fully extended.

d. Slowly start to lift up from the squat, until your legs are fully extended, squeeze your back and pull your elbows to your sides.

e. Remember that you are moving slowly to a three count, so it is one one thousand, two one thousand, three one thousand on the way down, pause for a beat, then the same speed as you return.

f. Inhale on the way down, exhale on the way up.

g. Make sure that you don't lose your posture, as shoulders should always stay back to stay long and lean.

h. As you lift up, focus on squeezing both your glutes and your back muscles.

NOTE: Don't allow momentum to take over. That is why I want you to move slowly through each repetition. Momentum is the enemy when your goal is successful, metabolism-enhancing strength training.

Progression

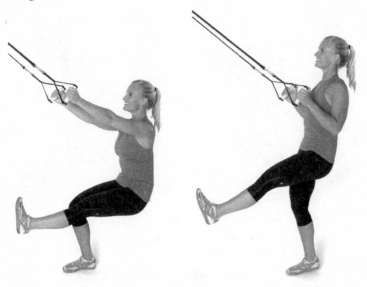

a. Start the exercise balancing on your left leg with your right leg extended.
b. Perform the same original exercise, in the same range of motion, but only on one leg.
c. Make sure to concentrate on the right glute when working the right leg and the left one when working the left leg.
d. To keep optimal form, dig in the heel of the working leg for stability.

This exercise gives you amazing, tight, sexy glutes!

Core

1. *Strap Roll-Outs*

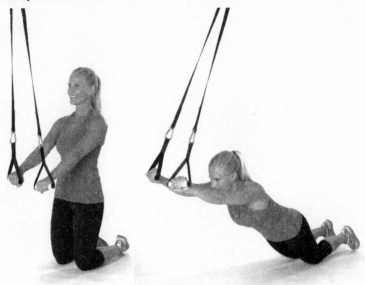

a. Start kneeling with your feet shoulder-width apart, arms extended down, shoulders back, and abs tucked, as pictured.

b. Slowly allow your body to shift forward, extending arms in front of you, like Superman.

c. Keep your abdominals tucked in to support your lower back at all times.

d. Remember that you are moving slowly to a three count, so it is one one thousand, two one thousand, three one thousand on the way out, pause for a beat, then the same speed as you return. Fight the urge to speed up this exercise.

f. Inhale on the way out, exhale on the way back.

g. You will also feel this exercise in your back, shoulders, and triceps, the back of your arms. Hourglass, here we come!

Progression – Standing

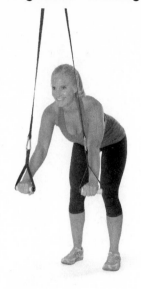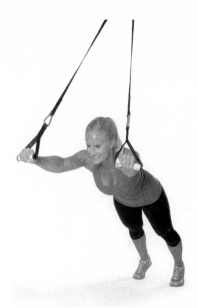

a. Start standing with your feet shoulder-width apart, arms extended down, shoulders back, hips hinged, and abs tucked, as pictured.

b. Again, slowly allow your body to shift forward, extending arms in front of you, like Superman.

c. This exercise is very intense. Don't be surprised if you can only perform 3-5 repetitions when you first attempt this progression.

2. *Standing Anti-Rotation Press*

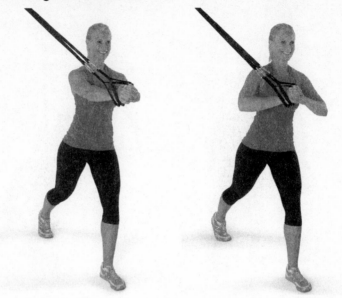

a. Start with left foot forward, right foot back, both toes facing forward, as pictured.

b. Place the right hand over both straps, then cup the left hand on top with arms fully extended.

c. Make sure that the tension is very taut at all times.

d. As you lean to the left, slowly bring your hands toward your chest, pause, then extend back out.

e. This exercise moves to a two count, so it is one one thousand, two one thousand on the way in, pause for a beat, then the same speed as you return.

f. Inhale as you bring your arms in, exhale as you return them to starting position.

g. Make sure to pull in your abdominals at all times.

h. Perform 10 repetitions and repeat on other side.

NOTE: If this is too easy, you are not leaning enough to the left.

Progression - Step closer to anchor point
(where you attached your straps to the door)

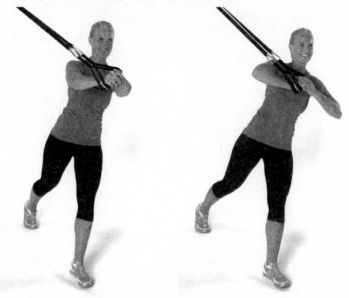

a. Perform the exact same exercise, same speed, but step closer to the anchor point.
b. This exercise becomes very difficult very quickly. Don't be surprised if you can only perform 3-5 repetitions when you first attempt this progression and find that you have to step farther away to finish the set.
c. Don't sacrifice form at any time, as this exercise shapes your core and promotes that hourglass figure you desire.

3. Prone Plank

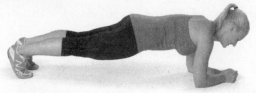

a. Start on your toes and elbows, as pictured.
b. The key is to keep your body parallel to the floor.
c. Hold this plank for 30 seconds, pause for 15 seconds, then repeat.
d. Keep your neck neutral by finding a spot on the floor in front of you and focusing on it.
e. Breathe comfortably throughout the exercise.
f. Make sure to really pull in your abdominals at all times.

NOTE: You will want to either raise or drop you hips, but don't because it takes tension off of your core, the muscle group we are activating.

1st Progression - Prone Plank in Straps

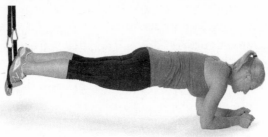

a. Start with your toes in straps, as pictured.
b. Once again, the key is to keep your body parallel to the floor.
c. Hold this plank for 30 seconds, pause for 15 seconds, then perform again.
d. Fight the urge to sway back and forth to challenge your core even more.

2nd Progression – Knee Tuck

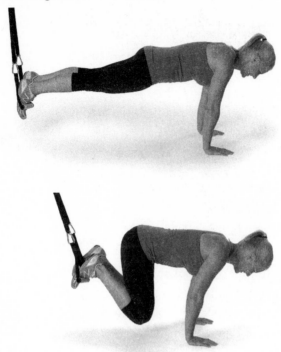

a. Start with your toes in straps, as pictured.

b. Once again, the key is to keep your body parallel to the floor.

c. This time, pull both knees in simultaneously until the knees are pointing straight down.

d. Make sure to keep your shoulders pulled back and your back flat.

NOTE: You will feel this in the abdominals, legs, shoulders, chest, and arms. Do I hear long and lean??

4. *Side Plank*

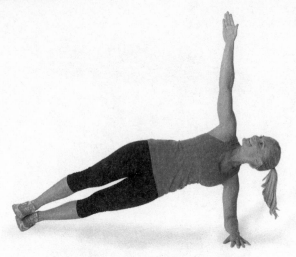

a. Start with your right foot on top of your left, resting on your left elbow, as pictured.

b. Your body is a perfectly straight line from feet to shoulders.

c. Extend your right arm up, fingers pointing straight up.

d. Pull your abdominals in and shoulders back at all times.

e. Hold for 30 seconds, rest for 15, then repeat on the same side.

f. Breathe comfortably throughout the exercise.

g. Repeat on other side.

Progression - Feet in Straps

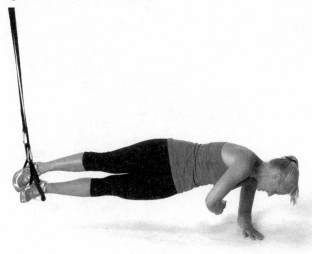

a. Start on your side, with both feet in straps, as pictured.

b. Once again, your body is a perfectly straight line from feet to shoulders.

c. Hold this plank for 30 seconds, pause for 15 seconds, then perform again.

d. Repeat on other side. FYI, feet in straps is HARD!!! Don't be surprised.

1. *Push-Up*

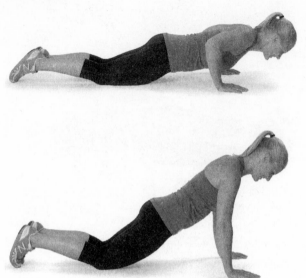

a. Start with your knees on the ground shoulder-width apart, and hands on the floor, slightly wider than shoulder-width.
b. Keep your abdominals tucked and shoulders back at all times.
c. Exhale as you press up for a three count, until your arms are almost fully extended—don't lock your elbows out—pause, then slowly inhale as you lower back to your starting position, approximately 2 inches from the floor.
d. Concentrate on your chest as you press up, as your goal is to engage the pectoral (chest) muscles, shoulders, and arms.
e. Make sure to keep your neck relaxed and in neutral position. Once again, focus on a point on the floor.

1st Progression – Full Push-Up

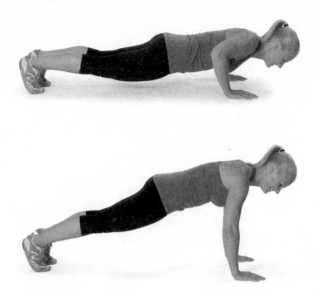

a. Start in the same position, except your knees are off of the ground, as pictured.

b. Your core, chest, and arms will be challenged given this progression.

c. Make sure to keep your abdominals tucked so that your body stays in a straight line from feet to shoulders, not putting tension on your lower back.

NOTE: These are not "boy" push-ups, these are "smart girl" push-ups!

2nd Progression – Push-Up with Feet in Straps

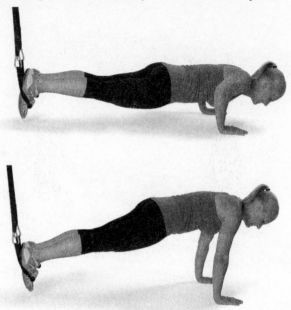

a. Start with both of your feet in individual straps.
b. Once again, your core, chest, and arms will be further challenged given this progression.
c. Don't allow your body to sway side to side. Fight with your
   core to keep your body in alignment.

2. One Leg Elevated Split Squat

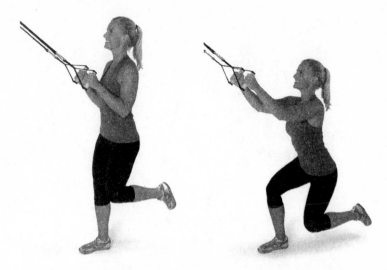

a. Start balancing on right foot, with your left leg bent, parallel to the floor, as pictured.

b. Hold the straps in each hand, palms facing each other, elbows at sides, and shoulders back (posture, posture, posture!).

c. Make sure that the tension is very taut in starting position.

d. Slowly start to lower your body down into a squat until your right hamstring is parallel to the floor.

e. Remember that you are moving slowly to a three count, so it is one one thousand, two one thousand, three one thousand on the way down, pause for a beat, then the same speed as you return.

f. Inhale on the way down, exhale on the way up.

g. Make sure to pull in your abdominals at all times.

h. Also, make sure that you are feeling the tension in your back and shoulders from the weight of your body against the tension of the strap.

Progression - One Leg in Strap

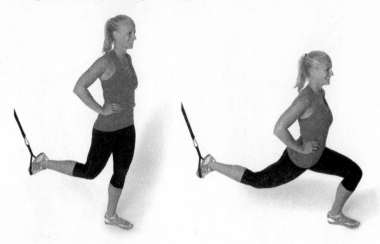

a. Start by placing your right leg in the strap, balancing on your left leg, as pictured.

b. Slowly extend your right leg behind you, as you perform a one-legged squat with the left leg.

c. Maintain good posture at all times and don't allow your body to lean forward.

NOTE: If you are feeling unstable, place a chair in front of you for guidance.

3. *Inverted Back Row*

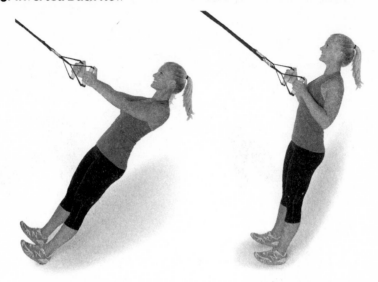

a. Start with your feet shoulder-width apart, shoulders back, and abs tucked.

b. Place your hands in the straps with palms facing each other and lean back with legs straight but not locked.

c. Make sure that the tension is very taut when your arms are fully extended.

d. Slowly start to pull your elbows to your sides, squeezing your shoulder blades together.

e. Remember that you are moving slowly to a three count, so it is one one thousand, two one thousand, three one thousand on the way up, pause for a beat, then the same speed as you return.

f. Inhale on the way up, exhale on the way back.

g. Make sure that you don't lose your posture, as shoulders should always stay pulled back. Posture is a Petite's BFF!

Progression – Step closer to anchor point

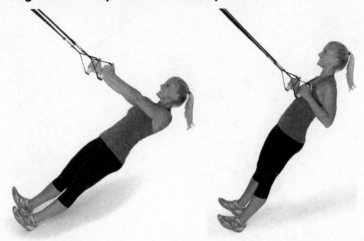

a. Move your feet closer to the anchor point. This adjustment will create far more tension on your back and arms.
b. Be aware of your neck alignment. Stare directly at your anchor point.
c. To keep optimal form, dig in the heels for stability.

4. Lateral Bounding (Speed Skaters)

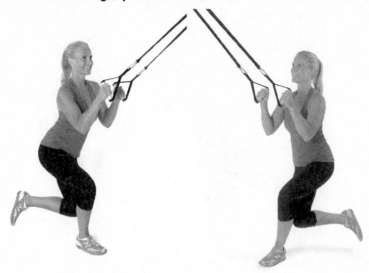

a. Start balancing on your right leg, left leg behind you parallel to the floor, as pictured.

b. Place each hand in individual straps, palms facing each other, with elbows slightly bent.

c. Make sure the straps are very taut when you are squatting to the right in your starting position.

d. Quickly jump to the left side, landing and performing a one-legged squat.

e. Unlike most of the exercises in this program, you are moving quickly from side to side as you are shocking your muscles and heart simultaneously, boosting your metabolism.

f. Breathe comfortably throughout the exercises.

g. Perform 10 repetitions on each leg alternating from side to side.

h. Maintain proper form throughout each repetition.

Progression - Simply jump farther from side to side

5. *Shoulder Press*

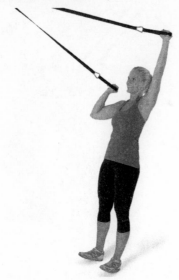

a. Start with your feet shoulder-width apart, shoulders back, and abs tucked.

b. Place one strap in each hand, palms facing forward, hands at ear height, and lean back slightly.

c. Make sure the tension of the straps is taut when your arms are in starting position.

d. Slowly extend the left arm up, keeping the right arm in starting position.

e. Remember that you are moving slowly to a three count, so it is one one thousand, two one thousand, three one thousand on the way down, pause for a beat, then the same speed as you return.

f. Exhale on the way up, inhale on the way down.

g. Alternate arms, performing one repetition with the left, followed by one repetition with the right.

h. Make sure you keep leaning back, maintaining tension on the muscles. If it's not hard, you are not leaning enough!

Progression

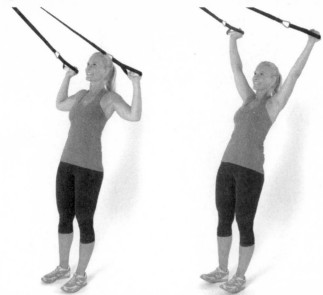

a. Assume starting position with both hands at ear height.

b. This time, press both arms up simultaneously.

c. Continue to lean back. Be aware of your neck alignment and stare directly at your anchor point.

d. To keep optimal form, dig in your heels for stability.

6. *Single-Leg Dead Lift*

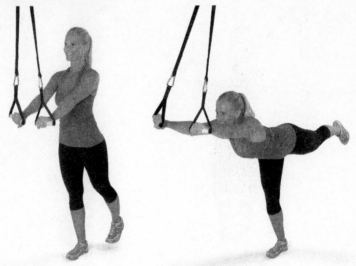

a. Start balancing on your right leg, with your left leg extended behind you, toe touching the floor, as pictured.

b. Place one strap in each hand, palms facing down with arms extended in front of you.

c. Make sure the tension of the straps is taut when your arms are extended in starting position.

d. Slowly start to lower your upper body as you extend the left leg straight back until your upper body and extended leg are parallel to the floor.

e. Remember that you are moving slowly to a three count, so it is one one thousand, two one thousand, three one thousand on the way down, pause for a beat, then the same speed as you return.

f. Inhale on the way down, exhale on the way up.

g. Make sure to pull in your abdominals at all times.

h. You will feel this exercise in the arms, core, glutes, and balancing leg.

Progression

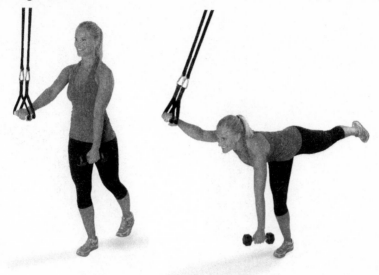

a. Assume starting position with right arm in both straps, left arm holding a weight (start with 5 lbs and progress accordingly).

b. As you bring your upper body and extended left leg parallel to the floor, extend the right arm while the left arm extends straight to the floor with the weight, as pictured.

c. It is very important to keep your back flat and extend your right arm forward and left leg back to optimize intensity and results.

7. Vertical Pull-Up

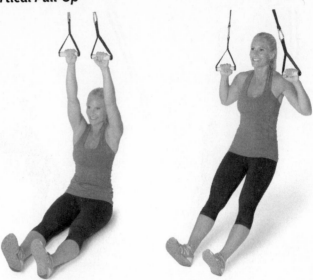

a. Start seated on floor, legs extended shoulder-width apart, abdominals tucked.

b. Place one strap in each hand with palms facing forward and extend arms straight up.

c. Make sure the tension is taut when your arms are up. Adjust straps accordingly.

d. Slowly start to pull your elbows to your side as you raise your body up until your hands are at shoulder height.

e. Remember that you are moving slowly to a three count, so it is one one thousand, two one thousand, three one thousand on the way up, pause for a beat, then the same speed as you return.

f. Exhale on the way up, inhale on the way down.

g. Make sure to pull in your abdominals at all times.

h. You will feel this exercise in your arms, back, and core.

Progression – One Leg Up

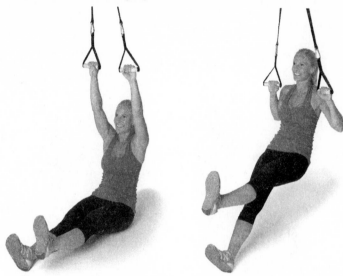

a. Assume the same starting position except the left leg is slightly raised off the floor and extended.

b. Dig your right heel in and slowly raise your body up, keeping your left leg up and extended.

c. It is very important to fight balance using your core, as that increases the intensity and results of the exercise.

8. Squat Jumps

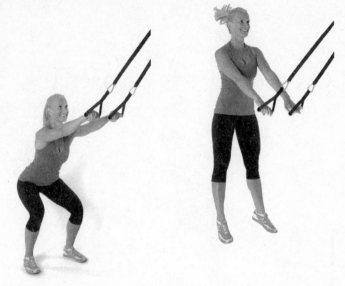

a. Start with your feet shoulder-width apart, shoulders back, and abs tucked.
b. With one strap in each hand, palms facing down, squat down until your hamstrings (backs of your legs) are parallel with the floor.
c. Make sure the tension is taut when your arms are extended as you squat.
d. Rapidly leap up in the air, pressing your arms down to the floor for momentum.
e. This is a metabolic movement meant to shock your entire body.
f. Make sure you land lightly on your toes first and roll onto your heels.
g. Perform 20 reps of this exercise and realize you are jumping for joy as the workout is over!!!

CHAPTER 9 PARTNERING UP
There Is Strength in Numbers

In chapter 1, we considered a research study that looked at the common denominators of people who had lost more than thirty pounds and have kept it off longer than three years. Every single part of that study correlates to what I have been doing with clients, both Petite and Non-Petite, for years. The sixth behavior noted in that study was: Establish a support system. Another study done at the University of Pittsburgh School of Medicine found that after ten months, 66 percent of those with a weight-loss buddy kept their weight off, versus 24 percent who went it alone. If you work the math of that research, you realize that you have over two and a half times *greater* chance of success when you "buddy up."

In this chapter, we'll look at how you can choose an appropriate partner and create a positive support system that will help you:

- Adjust your belief system

- Lose weight

- Stay totally full and ward off *all* hunger

- Experience, for the first time, a "reconfiguration"

Finding the Right Partner

My goal is to help you identify one team member who can help you deal with your beliefs and behaviors. To get you started, here are two questions I want you to ask yourself:

1. Do I have a very specific supportive person—spouse, partner, family member, or BFF—to rely on in my quest to be a leaner, sexier me?

2. How have people responded to me in the past when I attempted a weight-loss program?

The first question is a tough one for some to answer. You truly have to dig down and think, "Who can I count on with regard to this issue?" Notice that I didn't ask you to consider who you can count on in general, since you may have a terrific spouse or BFF who is great in most categories, but is not a help when it comes to resisting the baked ziti with butter-laden garlic bread followed by a tiramisu chaser on most Friday nights.

The research on this subject goes both ways. A Gallup poll conducted for *USA Today* and what used to be called *Discovery Health* (now called *OWN* and owned by Oprah Winfrey) found that:

57 percent said it would be a help to partner with a relative or friend.

68 percent said that their circle of friends has done more to help them succeed.

34 percent had problems with how they were treated by their circle of friends and relatives as they tempted them, teased them, and tried to derail their plans to exercise.

The first two bullet points are confirmed by Thomas Wadden, a weight-loss expert at the University of Pennsylvania School of Medicine, who states: "My experience is that partners want to help their loved one lose weight because they know it's important to the loved one." He goes on to say that "it's the exception rather than the rule that your partner is going to feel threatened by your weight loss and try to undermine your efforts."[1]

My experience is that your partner will either be somewhat supportive or deeply opposed to your weight-loss goals. The somewhat supportive partner will let you take the time to exercise and agree to keep high-calorie food out of the house, but this person generally is a bust in a social/restaurant setting when they feel you should both go ahead and "reward" yourselves since you have been "good" all week at home. Remember, for Petites, one big splurge dinner can take one week of diet and exercise to work off—just to get you back to square one. This spouse or significant other truly wants you to succeed, but also wants you both to have a good time and is conflicted or confused as to how to give you what you really need.

The other category of spouse or significant other can be very tough. He is probably also overweight and *loves* to eat and drink and avoid exercise. He really likes you as an eating and drinking buddy and doesn't want to hurt you, but also doesn't want to make changes in his own behavior. This makes it a real "mine field" when eating in or out together and in social settings. You have a few options:

1. Simply start to cook with fewer calories and see if your partner notices. If he does, explain; if he doesn't, just ride it out.

2. Place all Addies on the side so that you don't get hit with the added calories, but your partner still gets what he wants. That's a compromise that most people don't object to.

3. Choose restaurants that serve the type of food that keeps you on plan, but has options that he will enjoy—did I hear steak house?

4. Discuss your needs and compromise on what you will have in the house and how you will deal with that issue and with eating out. If you present it in a non-threatening manner, I don't think you will meet with much push-back.

I actually think a combination of all four of these suggestions makes the most sense, as you will have covered all the bases and

I have used the expression "The Buy-In" for years when it comes to weight loss. For women, especially Petites, you just want to get back down to a manageable weight that you enjoy. You also want to feel great. After Diane Sawyer lost her weight, people would ask her: "How do you stay on the plan now that you have lost all the weight?" Diane responded: "Look, sure I like the way I look, but the added energy I feel is amazing and keeps me on the eating and exercise plan." Energy was Diane's "Buy-in." For men, I find that an improved golf score provides a huge buy-in. When I tell a man that I can shave significant strokes off his game if he follows my plan of eating and exercising right, he bites—sometimes so hard that many of them have been hooked for life and their golf games have never been better. Try giving some thought to what could hook your partner. You might even try more sex. That seems to work with a lot of women I know.

will establish ground rules. Give it a try. Remember, you have nothing to lose—but weight. Besides, your behavior may start to rub off and then you will have a much more amenable partner.

You actually do have one other option—say nothing. Once again, lead by example, but have your guard up. This option is going to require that you have a lot of strength to ward off temptation *and* to deal with a person constantly asking why you aren't eating something.

Peer Review

Almost 100 percent of the time, I would urge you to choose a weight-loss buddy who is outside of your primary relationship. The biggest reason is that you most likely love your spouse or significant other because they *don't* make your weight an issue. They support and love you as you are. But that is not going to help you knock the weight off and adjust your belief and behavior to make it happen.

According to Adam Shafran, an exercise physiologist, chiropractor, and host of the Internet radio show *Dr. Fitness and the Fat Guy*, "Most people put all their effort into finding the right diet or exercise program but don't put any energy into creating a support and accountability system, and too often, that's where the devil lies."[2]

I speak all over the country on weight loss, enhanced health, anti-aging, and related topics. About three to four times a year, I am coupled with another very well-known speaker, Marshall Goldsmith. It's a big honor to be paired with Marshall, as he is an *über-*speaker (he can command what I call the "Clinton rates"), a Fortune 100 business coach, and the author of dozens of bestselling books on leadership, success, and management. Marshall taught me about what he calls "Peer Review," a concept that works perfectly for weight loss. Here is how it works.

Identify a person that you respect, who also possesses good ability to follow up, and shares a similar desire to lose weight (another reason why your primary relationship may not be the best choice). If you already know that someone is a little flaky—like someone who tries a new diet every other week—move on. The person you choose does *not* have to be a good friend. Just pick someone you trust who also has a desire to lose weight. You are going to follow up with this person on a monthly, weekly, or—my personal recommendation—daily basis. Here are the questions you are going to ask your Peer Review partner:

- Did you weigh yourself today?

- Did you keep a food journal yesterday?

- Were you active for sixty to ninety minutes yesterday?

- Did you perform your interval-based strength training for thirty-one minutes yesterday?

- Did you sleep seven to eight hours last night?

The only acceptable response by your partner to these questions is "yes" or "no."

The only acceptable response from you to these "yes" or "no" answers is "thank you."

You then switch roles and proceed under the same rules.

You each record—in a journal, on your computer, on your cell phone, whatever—the responses you received from your partner. It should become immediately apparent that the more "yes" answers you receive, the more weight your partner is losing. If your partner is not losing weight, then he or she (yes, you may use a man as your partner) is either lying or something else is going on. Again, my experience is that the more frequently you conduct this review, the more weight you will lose—and the more weight you will keep off. This "review" should go on for a long enough time, even after you have lost all your weight, to make sure that you are now holding yourself accountable and don't require the input of your partner.

What I like about Peer Review is that your reviewer holds you accountable. In the personal fitness-training business, I have always preached to my team that your #1 goal is to hold your client accountable for his or her actions. So frequently, clients start to complain and we hear comments like: "I'm not losing weight"; or "Your program doesn't work"; or "I'm going to quit." I am always quick to say: "Why aren't you losing weight? Are you on the program? Why say you are going to quit when you never really started?" That generally leads to a pause, a pained look, and a long talk about what we are *supposed* to be doing together. We talk about it in our initial consultation. We talk about it constantly. I hold my clients accountable at each and every session, and that is one of the reasons I am able to achieve such significant results the vast majority of the time.

According to a study conducted by Stanford University, small "nudging" like a phone call, whether from a real person or just a computer, proved to increase the number of minutes the participants exercised, although the "real person" results were higher.[3] Given that your partner is a real person and that you are being held responsible for, not just exercise, but overall activity, food (remember, weight loss is 75 percent diet and 25 percent exercise), and sleep, the odds are even greater that you will achieve your goal.

This is why I am also vehement about daily weigh-ins. You need to see the scale each and every day to know if you are actually on a trajectory to lose weight, maintain weight, or gain weight. All three results are data—although the third is a hard one to swallow. But, let's face it, you are swallowing *something* if the scale is going up. Use this data to your advantage.

Choosing someone for your partner is your first step. He or she doesn't have to be a Petite, as being petite is not essential for your success. I recommend working with your partner for one month. See what it is like to be held accountable, document your success, and *don't lie*! Why lie to yourself and to someone who is truly trying to help you deal with a tough issue? You only corrupt the respect you have for yourself and the respect you have for your partner.

Going Public

After you have that first month under your belt, you have to do what I urged my readers to do in *The Business Plan for the Body*. You have to "go public." It's time to tell the world that you are in the weight-loss business and plan on losing weight.

Yep, you have to let *everyone* know—your family members, both at home and your extended family, your co-workers, your friends, your book-club buddies—whoever you come in contact with on a regular basis who may observe that you are looking and behaving differently. This is important, as you need to make a few adjustments, like taking inventory of your family members and friends. According to James Fowler, Ph.D. and professor at the University of California at San Diego, and Nicholas Christakis, M.D., Ph.D. and sociology professor at Harvard, "Having a buddy who packs on the pounds makes you 57 percent more likely to do so yourself." That is a *huge* figure—57 percent. Fowler goes on to say: "Consciously or unconsciously, people look to others when deciding what and how much to eat, and how much weight is too much."[4] You will find great support from those who are already at a more comfortable weight, but be prepared to deal with the others. Don't forget, 68 percent of our present population is overweight.

I want to stay on this topic for a moment. I observe, *all the time*, that circles of friends are either really working on their weight or they are not. I see it at my kids' school, at parties, and at stores. Generally, the women roving in packs appear to be closer in weight. Sure, you occasionally see a few more overweight, but they are clearly in the minority. Look at your own circle of friends and family members. You may see a trend.

If you don't believe me, here is what three experts have to say on the subject of friends and weight loss:

> John McGrail, a Los Angeles clinical hypnotherapist and behavioral expert, says, "Human beings are hard-wired to resist change, so it's not uncommon to encounter some resistance whenever change occurs."

> Christian Holle, Ph.D. and Assistant Professor of Psychology at William Paterson University, adds, "In some ways, your weight loss becomes a symbol of their inability to accomplish their goals, so they may begin to act resentful—or even mean—oftentimes without even realizing they are doing so."

> Warren Huberman, Ph.D. and psychologist who counsels patients in weight loss, finishes with the fact that "You may find that [friends] are suddenly excluding you from activities, saying mean things, taunting you about your new body or even your new clothes."[5]

This issue of how women respond to another's weight loss is truly important. I had a lovely young woman in her early thirties

> **In this day and age,** with 68 percent of our population overweight, those of us at a more appropriate weight are in the minority. We actually get picked on. I do, but that clearly is a function of my business. Unfortunately, so do others. Isn't it ironic that we covet the skinny celebrities and can't wait to hear about the next "quick-fix" diet, but then we criticize those who do succeed at losing weight? That is why the people around you are so influential, either in a positive or negative way.

who lost over 100 pounds. That's an amazing accomplishment. Unfortunately, the women at her church—that's right, her place of worship—were horrible to her. They actually went up to her and made comments like: "I bet you think you are better than me now." Ouch. You go through all the time and effort to lose weight and then get slammed for it. Have your antenna up. Be prepared and, when all else fails, smile!

Look, I get this all the time. Overweight people say to me, "I bet you don't eat that," as they point to the mammoth-size cupcakes at a birthday party that no adult or child has any business eating. I politely say: "Oh, I would love one, but then I'd have to cut way back at dinner tonight and I just don't want to have to do that."

Please don't ignore this issue. I am purposefully packing this chapter with research and case studies in addition to my own experiences to prove to you that your environment and the people in that environment are as critical to your success as your belief system. They are influencing your beliefs. Be aware of that fact and be prepared.

Another adjustment you have to make is to keep food off the table. Cornell University researchers found that serving yourself elsewhere—for instance, at the kitchen counter or stove—resulted in 35 percent less food being consumed than when it just sat on the table. You *have* to get the food off the table and out of your sight.[6] Since I have talked about children in the past, I think it is also smart to say that, if you are serving the whole family, everyone benefits when you get the food off the table.

This also keeps you from picking. I find picking to be a huge issue for many women—and one that really hits you as a Petite much harder than your taller friends. You don't have any idea how many calories you are "picking" at, so here's another idea for you. Every time you go to pick up a leftover chicken nugget (I hope it's baked!) from your child's plate or pop in that crust of bread or piece of leftover pizza (I hope it's made/ordered with less cheese and more veggies), put it in a Ziploc bag and throw it in the refrigerator. Do this for just three days. You won't believe the responses I got from clients who tried this in the past. Some said that they had to go to a second bag—in just three days! That alone may be a part of the reason why you are struggling with your weight. Picking counts and, by going back to the math, you will find that those pickings add up very fast.

Another step you can take is to beware of "Dining with Dames." According to a study by Meredith Young of McMaster University in Ontario, "women eat nearly 250 calories less when they dine with men, compared to when dining with other women."[7] The author theorizes that "subconsciously, women may feel that men will find them more attractive if they don't eat a lot." You should have your antenna up and activated when you are eating with other women.

And make sure that you keep temptation out of sight *and* out of mind.

Hunger and Your Brain

There was a recent article in the *Wall Street Journal* entitled "Eating to Live or Living to Eat" that talked about how the brains of the overweight and obese "light up" when they see, smell, or just hear of certain foods like sugary desserts. The researchers found that:

- Brain scans of the overweight and obese showed that they had stronger reactions to the image, smell, or sound of certain foods—generally fatty sweets like cake—than to leaner foods.

- Obese people stop responding to the hormone leptin, which I will explain in the next chapter with regard to sleep. Those individuals who were sleep-deprived showed diminished levels of leptin. If you recall, leptin is the hormone that tells your mind and body that you are getting full and helps you to push away from the table. The issue here is that obese bodies *are* producing leptin in larger quantities than their leaner counterparts, but the brains of these obese individuals stop taking its cue.

- Tempting food *does* stimulate the release of the "desire chemical" dopamine, and this happens in both obese and non-obese individuals. However, the obese appear in studies to possess fewer dopamine receptors. Therefore, they derive less pleasure from eating the sugary, fat-laden food and this sets them up to crave even more. It's a bit like the drug addict who could get high when they first experimented with drugs on a small dose. But over time, they require more and more to mimic the same response. It sounds to me as if the same is happening with food.

I have often had women tell me how full and uncomfortable they feel—"I am totally stuffed"—and then order dessert *and* pound

When we talk about the brain and weight loss,
the question is what came first—the overeating or the
brain's response to overeating? This is similar to how
people are developing type II diabetes because they are
repeatedly asking for that huge insulin response that
occurs after eating the wrong foods. After pumping out
so much more insulin than it planned, the pancreas
malfunctions. You blow it out.

The same thing may be occurring with your brain.
By lighting it up all the time with the temptation of the
wrong foods, your body starts saying "give me more,
give me more" and you crave these foods and need more
and more of them to feel satisfied. I've had clients who
said, whereas just a few years ago two or three cookies
would have done the trick, now they need five times that
many to get the same satisfaction. Stay tuned for more
research on this; I'm sure it will be forthcoming.

the cookies and chocolates sitting on the table as they drink three
cups of coffee that is actually half coffee, half cream. I don't need
to tell you the size of these women.[8]

I believe that you truly *must* do the following, at least for the
first twenty-one days of this plan:

- Remove all tempting food from the house. I mean all of it. I
  don't want to hear, "but the kids need crap in the house." No,
  they really don't. Load the house with fruit, vegetables, lean
  protein, and other things that are on your plan, and watch
  everyone benefit.

- Decline invitations to meals with people who will not be respectful of your needs. You don't need people around you who say, "Oh, you can cheat tonight with me." *No, no, no.* These are exactly the kind of people that will derail your success. Why is it that people feel they have the right to determine when you will cheat? Isn't that your choice? I actually urge you to call your hostess in advance and politely let her know that you are on a specific plan, and request that she please keep all Addie foods on the side and not mention that you are on a special eating plan unless you want to bring it up. People also feel compelled to say things like "Just so you know, my friend, Pamela, sitting over there, is on a diet." That puts the kibosh on the whole experience. You know who these women are. Avoid them until you are mentally and psychically ready.

- Jump in and decide what restaurant you are going to go to for meals. I have a few favorites in Chicago. One, which happens to be Oprah's favorite as well, RL, actually serves what they call "Jim Karas Chicken," which is chicken paillard (that's the pounded, thin breast) cooked without oil and with lots of lemon. Then I can have whatever steamed veggie I want (I generally try to stay in season for freshness) on the bottom. I love it; I eat it all the time. It fills me up and usually half the table orders it with me. Clients and friends in the restaurant actually hold their plates up and show me that they are eating my dish. It's simple. Remember, the steak house is your best friend. Visit it as often as possible.

And above all, watch for triggers. Now, this could apply to almost everything I have talked about in this chapter, since people, places, and situations can *all* be placed in the "trigger" category. I define a trigger as a "loss of control over eating." David Kessler,

M.D. and author of *The End of Overeating*, reports that triggers happen to "50 percent of the obese, 30 percent of the overweight and even 20 percent of those at healthy weight."[9] You need to be extremely aware of these triggers, as they generally lead to big splurges that pack the pounds on Petites. As I urged you before, *plan*. Download menus, ask—whatever it takes to keep the pounds off and you on your plan.

Now, this does not have to be forever. Just for twenty-one days, as most research indicates that it takes twenty-one days to break a habit. That's another reason why I made this Petite plan twenty-one days long.

CHAPTER 10

THE BAG OF TRICKS
Why Sleeping, Stress Relief, and Mind-Set Are So Important to Petites

In the introduction, I eluded to the small reductions in calories and the small increases in metabolism that make a *big* difference to Petites.

As much as I feel it is imperative that you follow my eating and exercise plan to the best of your ability, you must also keep these points in mind, as they will either minimize or totally derail your likelihood of success.

Sleep

Sleep is critically important to your successful weight loss. According to a study conducted by the American Cancer Society, the average American was sleeping eight hours a night in 1960 and is now sleeping, *on average*, 6.7 hours. I italicized *on average*, as I believe many people are sleeping far less than that in the classic urban and suburban, overscheduled, overstressed environment. Why is this so detrimental to Petites? Because sleep deprivation is directly linked to weight gain. Two critical hormones that regulate appetite and satiety—leptin and ghrelin—are adversely impacted by a lack of sleep.

Leptin, produced in fat cells, acts as an appetite regulator and assists you in pushing away from the table when you are physically full. Think of leptin as satiety's BFF. With leptin around, your satiety levels are firing away and your body properly responds to this very influential signal when it is full (except for those mentioned in the previous chapter who appear to be what is called "leptin-resistant"). In numerous studies, the moment participants were sleep-deprived, their leptin levels dropped, and this happened as quickly as in one night. Therefore, the researchers observed that participants ate more for no other reason than a lack of leptin, which was reduced by a lack of sleep.

Leptin levels also reduce the moment you go on a calorie-reducing diet, so if you are cutting calories, which is what I am urging you to do—although the calorie cycling will help to mitigate that drop—coupling that with sleep deprivation will cause your leptin levels to drop that much further. That is why sleep is so very important when you are on this plan and also why the calorie cycling works mentally *and* physically to ward off hunger, the enemy of all Petites.

Ghrelin, which is produced in the gastrointestinal tract, stimulates appetite. Think of ghrelin as the plant in the play/movie *Little Shop of Horrors*—the one that keeps saying "Feed me!" Researchers find there is an inverse relationship between sleep and ghrelin. When participants are sleep-deprived, their ghrelin levels elevate, which results in them eating more. Again, this happened almost immediately when participants were sleep-deprived.

Many studies have been conducted, but the University of Chicago and Stanford University studies both conclusively proved that less sleep correlated to more weight. And the less participants slept, the more they weighed. It showed a perfect inverse relationship.

Let's go back to our belief system. The vast majority of overweight people I come across do not believe in this sleep/weight relationship. They have yet another flawed belief system. They tell me that they have to stay up to get things done or that they don't need that much sleep or that they have trained themselves to operate on less sleep.

My response to them, respectively, is: "No you don't"; "Yes, you do"; and "No, you haven't."

When you stay up to get things done, you operate at a much lower mental and physical capacity the next day, as you are exhausted. Your mind is not as sharp, your attention and memory functions slow down, and the speed at which you think is diminished. And, quite frankly, you generally feel like crap. You do not feel like moving around (which we have established is critically important), nor do you have any desire to exercise with intensity (ditto—critically important). Oh, you do one thing better than you did when you were properly rested—you eat! You eat because your hormones are out of whack. What do the vast majority of people do when they are sleep-deprived? They eat to try to stay awake. Think about that for a moment. Your energy levels are weakened as a result of insufficient sleep, so you add insult to injury by eating more, which also depletes precious energy. I'm surprised you can even move around, let alone get anything done.

The research is unanimous: you require seven to eight hours of sleep each night. Once again, your flawed belief system allows you to believe that sleep deprivation is a positive, when I am here to tell you it is a serious negative, especially as it applies to weight loss.

Researchers at Columbia University in New York City found that:

> **Sleep enhances testosterone.** *Testosterone is criti-*
> *cally important to you, as a Petite, since it is essential for*
> *muscle growth (which I have established is a cornerstone*
> *of this plan), increased metabolism (ditto), sex drive (gotta*
> *love that), and energy. That newfound energy is going*
> *to give you the ability to change your belief system and*
> *stay strong around the wrong people or the wrong foods,*
> *make those smarter food choices, exercise with intensity,*
> *and move more in general.*[1]

- Those who slept only six hours a night had a 23 percent greater chance of obesity.

- Those who slept only five hours a night had a 50 percent greater chance of obesity.

- Those who slept only four hours or fewer had a 73 percent greater chance of obesity.[2]

And no, you have not effectively learned to operate on less sleep. Your body has simply stopped asking for it. This is the exact same thing that happens to people who no longer drink water. Their bodies just stop asking for it, since they didn't give them any. Ditto with skipping breakfast and saying "But I'm not hungry." You aren't hungry because your body just stopped asking for food in the morning. It makes sense, if you think about it. You can train your body to react positively to what you do repeatedly, and you can train your body to react negatively to what you do repeatedly. It's a two-way street.

If you are not regularly sleeping seven to eight hours a night, something is terribly wrong and you need to keep a log of when you go to bed each night and when you get up each morning. That is why the sleep question was a part of your Peer Review. By making sleep a priority, you dramatically increase your odds of success at weight loss.

I also urge you to develop what I suggest in *The 7-Day Energy Surge*—a "sleep strategy." Here is how you develop your strategy:

- Determine what time you will get up tomorrow morning.

- Now, work backward to ascertain what time you need to be asleep tonight (notice I said asleep, not in bed) to get between seven and eight hours of sleep.

- Determine what helps put you to sleep. Is it a hot shower or bath to relax your mind and body? Should you light candles? Lavender, chamomile, and ylang-ylang are believed to be sleep inducers.

- No computer in bed thirty minutes before you plan on falling asleep. You may watch TV, but please keep to a rerun of *Everyone Loves Raymond* or *Seinfeld*. Don't watch *Bride of Chucky* and expect to fall into blissful sleep after you have stressed your mind and body to the max.

- Work both ends. What you do when you wake up first thing in the morning helps to determine when you fall asleep at night. When you wake up, first perform your deep breathing for five to ten minutes (you will learn about it in a moment), then turn all the lights on or open your drapes/shades, or both. Light tells your brain "we're up and ready to rock" and that will enhance what is called your circadian rhythm—which is simply your "wake/sleep" cycle. Similarly, when it starts to get dark, your body hormonally says to itself, "we are going to go to bed soon" and starts to produce melatonin to prepare your mind and body for sleep. You literally control how your mind and body behave later in the evening by what you do first thing in the

> ***Don't eat to music with a fast beat,*** *as it may make you eat and drink more.*

morning. And the hormone melatonin detoxifies harmful, cancer-causing free radicals (we've talked about them a number of times), creates more fighter cells (we want them to stay healthy), and may even boost the power of vitamin C. Those are big reasons to get that hormone pumping at night.[3]

- Go to bed and get up within the same thirty minutes every day. I do this 90 percent of the time and my most successful Petites keep a pretty tight schedule. Again, this optimizes your hormones to your advantage and comes with the added plus of pretty impressive energy levels.

Petites, please understand that your smaller stature makes you more vulnerable to hormonal imbalance. Therefore, do everything in your power to enable your body to shed the weight. Getting to bed is clearly only a win-win proposition—or should I say lose-lose proposition when it comes to weight! There are lots of tricks to give your body the sleep it needs. One is to eliminate stress.

Stress

I don't have to tell you that stress levels are off the charts these days, and I don't really see things changing that much for the better in the near future. I so strongly dislike people who say things like "relax," or "don't take things so seriously," or "it will all be fine." That type of response did nothing but infuriate me when I was running at full "stress throttle" in the past. But, what you can do is rely upon some effective stress-reducing techniques like deep breathing, listening to music, or turning off the technical "chatter."

I frequently start my day with deep breathing. I lie in bed, place one hand on my diaphragm, and then slowly breathe in through my nose. You place your hand on your diaphragm because you want to feel your lungs fill up with air. So frequently, we are pulling our stomachs in or wearing something too tight that constricts our breathing. Instead, I want you to use this time to let your lungs fill up freely and your stomach push out comfortably. That's the goal of this type of exercise.

I start by breathing in through my nose for a count of four—one one thousand, two one thousand, three one thousand, four one thousand. Hold for those same four counts; then exhale through your mouth for the same four counts. Try to go for an extra "one thousand" and see if you can get up to eight or nine counts. I find that if I do this for just five to ten minutes each morning, I start my day out right. It just centers me to breathe, and I urge you to do the same.

This also works at any time during the day. Sometimes, when I am waiting to pick up my kids or standing in line, I also work on my breathing. It's so easy and all the research concurs that deep breathing can significantly reduce stress hormones. I recall a statistic that said that just ten minutes of deep breathing can reduce stress hormones by 44 percent. That's a huge reduction that may make a big difference in your weight loss.

Music also has tremendous stress-reducing powers that include helping you fall asleep. One research study showed that listening to soothing music for just forty-five minutes before going to bed helped breathing slow down (and slowing down generally indicates deeper breath, which is the goal), helped people fall asleep faster, and also resulted in deeper sleep, which is the most rejuvenating.[4] Another study used high school students (talk about stress!) and urged them to listen to relaxing music for one month. Seventy-four percent said they were able to fall asleep within ten minutes. That's fast.[5]

I also love music that can pep you up. I know that I cannot work out without my iPod blaring in my ears, and there is research that says that the pumped-up music actually enables you to work out harder (that's key!) and longer (which is not as important as the intensity).

Another stress-reducing technique is to light candles. Researchers recommend lighting peppermint candles, as the minty aroma stimulates alertness, which may distract you from making poor snack choices. When you are feeling stressed, just light a candle, breathe, and turn on some soothing music. Talk about the one-two-three punch for reducing stress!

I also feel the opposite way about the power of candles when it comes to falling asleep. I strongly recommend that you dim the lights about an hour before you plan on falling asleep. Notice that I didn't say "before you get into bed," but actually before you turn out the lights and fall asleep. I believe that candles possess healing powers that let your mind and body shut down. Therefore, they help you "wind down" and tell your body "we are getting ready for bed." Remember what I keep saying—you tell your body, through your actions and beliefs, what to do. By telling your body that you are getting ready for bed, you make your body behave accordingly.

And what better way to relieve stress than to get a massage. I am a huge fan of massage, whether you get one from a trained professional, a partner or friend, or give one to yourself. Massage brings blood to your muscles, which helps them repair, especially when you are performing strength training. It also relaxes your muscles. This will help to de-stress your entire body. If done the right way, you can massage the area where your chest muscles attach to your shoulder muscles to help improve posture.

Again, as a Petite, your body gets hit that much harder by an influx of stress hormones because of your size. Think of two fireplaces, one big and one small, with the same amount of wood and flame. Clearly the smaller fireplace is going to heat up more than the larger one, because the fire is confined to a smaller space. The flame is that much closer to the brick or stone. That small fireplace is you and that flame is the stress response in your body. That's why, when stress literally "lights you up," your body and mind get hit that much harder.

CONCLUSION: IT'S YOUR CHOICE

I chose to close this book with a simple concept: It's your choice. It's your choice whether you want to live your life in your present body or make a change. This book has taught you a number of lessons that only you can choose to apply to your life.

First, I taught you that *selfish is good!* Truer words have never been spoken, especially for Petites. You have to own that and understand, once again, that, when you are selfish, *everyone* benefits.

Next, you learned about metabolism—your weapon of mass reduction. You have to rock it. Come on, as a Petite you can choose to rock that metabolism and it will reward you with weight loss. That's a great payoff if you ask me.

From The Math you learned that small changes can result in pounds dropping off—for good. These changes are sometimes tough to swallow, but necessary. You can't eat like the big people, but you can look amazing and be lean and strong. It's the card you were dealt—not the Jack of Spades, but the Queen of Hearts. I will even go so far as to say that it's the Queen of *Lean* Hearts. You can choose to play that card.

Then you learned the rules of the Eating Game: Chow big to stay small. I've given you a lot of meal options to choose from. I love to eat, don't get me wrong. But even I have to be careful at six feet tall. You just have to be that much more aware.

My eating plan gives you many choices. You must choose why, where, when, and what you will eat. Just follow the plan. You have only one thing to lose—*weight!*

The chapter on eating out will help you make the right choices to take control of The Monster. I love to eat out and so should you. You can enjoy eating out and still stay totally on plan—and have fun. Enjoy. Just be ready to make the right choices in each and every situation, which I feel I have prepared you for.

And remember to look out for liquid calories—Public Enemy #1. Just know they are poison. Truly. With the exception of some low-fat milk and wine, you really should eliminate them. Is a glass of juice really worth it? Your choice.

Choose to make exercise your BFF. You will totally shrink if you give it a try.

Make a good choice when you partner up. Yes, there is strength in numbers. You may have done this with or without success in life. Trust me, when it comes to weight loss, there is no downside to choosing the right partner and having that person help you drop big pounds.

These lessons will all help you make the right choices to achieve your weight-loss goal and accomplish your first "recomposition." After that, your biggest problem will be losing your voice in the clothing store when you keep saying to the saleswoman: "Don't you have this in a *smaller* size?"

ACKNOWLEDGMENTS

As this is my fifth book, I find that the dedication and acknowledgments actually become harder, not easier. With a first book, you basically thank the people who helped you get published in the first place. As you move forward, you think a little bit more about "who really helped me to make this happen?"

So, here is my "happen" list:

To my team of trainers in Chicago and New York, thank you for proudly raising the bar on the "Karas" brand. I know it's not always easy pumping out session after session, but you clearly do it with integrity, honesty, and true passion. You also rock the Jim Karas Personal Training uniform, which inspires me to take my own body to the next level . . . and I'm 50.

To their leader, Phil Chung, whom I call "Philippe." You teach me a lot as a leader, a father (he has a brood of three children under the age of eighteen months), a partner (along with his amazing wife, Abby), and a person. The expression "the sky is the limit" clearly applies to you. Let's keep working together to get there, in every respect.

I must also give a "shout out" to Kristen Freiburger, who is not only our director of marketing but is also our Petite fitness model in chapter 8. I hope Kristen finally marries Chris Hiller, her boyfriend, who skillfully helped me with the meal plan, shopping list, and recipes. And a second "shout out" to Andrew Gallagher, who helped me create this exercise program.

Next, to my BFF, Cynthia Costas Cohen, MFA. Not only did she coauthor my last book, *The 7-Day Energy Surge*, but she is also a guide / sister / brilliant therapist to me in life and has no problem saying to me regularly, with all good intentions, "What the fu&&%k were you thinking?"

Finally, to my two personal "Petites," Olivia and Evan, who also happen to be my children.

Olivia, I marvel at your commitment to your gymnastics (she's nationally ranked, so I'm allowed to brag) and equally to your friends, your school, and to life in general. With the slight exception of when you are a "fishwife" to your brother and me (can you please give us a break every now and then?) you bring me not only joy, but great admiration. I wish I had your confidence and focus when I was your age.

Evan, right now, you aspire to be an artist, actor, soccer player, and circus performer. That's an ambitious list. While I may not be that keen on the circus choice, I do respect your passion, conviction, and "hey, this is me" attitude. I only hope you let me know before college if circus performing is your true passion!!!

NOTES

Introduction

1. Marc Ambinder, "Beating Obesity," *The Atlantic*, May 2010, accessed January 10, 2011, http://www.theatlantic.com/magazine/archive/2010/04/beating-obesity/8017/.
2. Amy Paturel, "The ABCs of Slim," *Women's Health*, February 2008, 104.
3. *International Journal of Obesity*, 33, 727-735 (July 2009), doi:10.1038/ijo.2009.76.
4. Kevin Helliker, "Food May Be Addicting for Some," *Wall Street Journal*, accessed April 5, 2011, http://online.wsj.com/article/SB10001424052748703712504576243192495912186.html.

Chapter 1: Selfish Is Good!

1. "Beliefs Impact Behavior," *Johns Hopkins Bloomberg School of Public Health*, December 7, 2006, accessed January 10, 2011, http://www.jhsph.edu/publichealthnews/articles/2006/hbs_fishbein.html.
2. James Hill, Ph.D., and Rena Wing, Ph.D., "The National Weight Control Registry," *The Permanente Journal*, Summer 2003: Vol. 7, No. 3, accessed January 10, 2011, http://xnet.kp.org/permanentejournal/sum03/registry.html.

Chapter 2: Metabolism

1. "Basal metabolic rate," *Wikipedia*, accessed January 10, 2011, http://en.wikipedia.org/wiki/Basal_metabolic_rate.
2. *American Journal of Epidemiology*, 2003, Jul 1; 158(1): 85-92.
3. John Cloud, "Why Exercise Won't Make You Thin," *Time*, accessed January 10, 2011, http://www.time.com/time/health/article/0,8599,1914857-4,00.html.
4. *British Journal of Nutrition* (2001), 85: 203-211.
5. Sharon Palmer, R.D., "Bold and Beautiful Spices for Health," *Environmental Nutrition*, August 2010: Vol. 33, No. 8: 1, 4.
6. "Sitting at Work All Day May Be Harmful, Erase Exercise Benefits," accessed January 10, 2011, http://www.wtae.com/r/22313482/detail.html.

Chapter 3: The Math

1. Deborah W. Kiel, Elizabeth A. Dodson, Raul Artal, Tegan K. Boehmer, Terry L. Leet, "Gestational Weight Gain and Pregnancy Outcomes in Obese

Women: How Much Is Enough?" *Obstetrics & Gynecology*, 110 (4) (2007): 752–758, accessed 3/15/2011, doi: 10.1097/01.AOG.0000278819.17190.87, http://journals.lww.com/greenjournal/fulltext/2007/10000/gestational_weight_gain_and_pregnancy_outcomes_in.5.aspx.

Chapter 4: The Eating Game

1. J. S. Vander Wal, A. Gupta, P. Khosla, N. V. Dhurandhar, "Egg breakfast enhances weight loss," *International Journal of Obesity*, October 2008; 32(10): 1545–1551.
2. Sharon Palmer, R.D. "Bold and Beautiful Spices for Health," *Environmental Nutrition*, August 2010: Vol. 33, No. 8: 1, 4.
3. Koh-Banerjee, Pauline, Eric B. Rimm, "Whole grain consumption and weight gain: a review of the epidemiological evidence, potential mechanisms and opportunities for future research," *Proceedings of the Nutrition Society* (2003); 62: 25–29.

Chapter 6: Eating Out

1. "Only 8% of Americans Eat Enough Fruits (Veggies—Even Worse)," *Fooducate Blog*, November 18th, 2010, accessed March 23, 2011, http://www.fooducate.com/blog/2010/11/18/only-8-of-americans-eat-enough-fruits-veggies-even-worse/.
2. Marian Burros, "Losing Count of Calories as Plates Fill Up," *New York Times*, April 2, 1997, accessed March 23, 2011, http://query.nytimes.com/gst/fullpage.html?res=9C06E0DA1F3AF931A35757C0A961958260&pagewanted=all.

Chapter 7: Liquid Calories

1. Kiyah J. Duffey and Barry M. Popkin, *Obesity*, November 2007, 15–11: 2739–2746.
2. "Beverage Consumption a Bigger Factor in Weight," *Johns Hopkins Bloomberg School of Public Health*, December 7, 2006, accessed January 10, 2011, http://www.jhsph.edu/publichealthnews/press_releases/2009/caballero_beverage_consumption.html.
3. Tom Hansen, "Know Your Daily Liquid Calorie Intake," *Women's Health Magazine*, accessed January 19, 2011, http://www.womenshealthmag.com/nutrition/liquid-sugar-intake.
4. S. H. Babey, M. Jones, H. Yu, H. Goldstein, "Bubbling over: soda consumption and its link to obesity in California," *Policy Brief UCLA Center for Health Policy Research*, 2009; 1–8.
5. Sharon P. Fowler, M.P.H. Abstract 1058-P, University of Texas Health Science Center School of Medicine.
6. Fowler, Abstract 1058-P.
7. M. Boschmann, J. Steiniger, U. Hille, J. Tank, F. Adams, A. M. Sharma, S.

Klaus, F. C. Luft, J. Jordan, "Water-induced thermogenesis," *Journal of Clinical Endocrinology and Metabolism*, 88: 6015–6019, 2003.

8. "Your Cup of Tea," *Men's Health*, March 2004: 48.
9. "Boil It Down," *Men's Health*, December 2005: 52.
10. "Drink This, Go Long," *Men's Health*, June 2005: 56.
11. Julija Josic, Anna T. Olsson, Jennie Wickeberg, Sandra Lindstedt, Joanna Hlebowicz, "Does green tea affect postprandial glucose, insulin and satiety in healthy subjects: a randomized controlled trial," *Nutrition Journal* 2010, 9:63, accessed 3/15/2011, doi: 10.1186/1475-2891-9-63, http://www.nutritionj.com/content/9/1/63.
12. "Antioxidant," Wikipedia, accessed January 10, 2011, http://en.wikipedia.org/wiki/Antioxidant.
13. S. G. Wannamethee, A. E. Field, G. A. Colditz, E. B. Rimm, "Alcohol intake and 8-year weight gain in women: a prospective study," *Obesity Research* 2004; 12(9): 1386–1396.

Chapter 8: Exercise

1. Jane E. Brody, "To Avoid 'Boomeritis,' Exercise, Exercise, Exercise," *The New York Times*, December 19, 2006, accessed December 12, 2011, http://www.nytimes.com/2006/12/19/health/19brody.html?pagewanted=all.
2. M. Wilson, "Diverse patterns of myocardial fibrosis in lifelong, veteran endurance athletes," *Journal of Applied Physiology*, June 2011, accessed December 12, 2011, http://www.ncbi.nlm.nih.gov/pubmed/21330616.
3. Gary Taubes, "The Scientist and the Stairmaster," *New York*, September 24, 2007, accessed December 12, 2001, http://nymag.com/news/sports/38001/index3.html.
4. R. W. Bryner, *Journal of the American College of Nutrition*, April 18, 1999, "Effects of resistance vs. aerobic training combined with an 800 calorie liquid diet on lean body mass and resting metabolic rate," http://www.ncbi.nlm.nih.gov/pubmed/10204826.

Chapter 9: Partnering Up

1. Nanci Hellmich, "Friends help carry the burden of dieting," *USA Today*, accessed February 8, 2011, http://www.usatoday.com/news/health/weightloss/2008-01-06-weight-loss-friends_N.htm.
2. Adam Shafran, "Benefits of Finding a Diet Buddy," *Web MD*, accessed February 8, 2011, http://www.webmd.com/diet/guide/choosing-weight-loss-buddy?page=3.
3. Kevin Helliker, "The Power of a Gentle Nudge," *Wall Street Journal*, accessed February 8, 2011, http://online.wsj.com/article/SB10001424052748704314904575250352409843386.html.
4. Courtney Rubin, "Lose the Weight: Are Your Friends a Fat Influence?"

Women's Health Magazine, accessed February 8, 2011, http://www.womens
healthmag.com/weight-loss/healthy-weight-loss.

5. Colette Bouchez, "Are They Jealous of Your New Body?" *MedicineNet,*
   accessed February 8, 2011, http://www.medicinenet.com/script/main/art.asp?
   articlekey=56031.

6. "Clear the Table," *Men's Health Magazine,* September 2010, 38.

7. M. E. Young, M. Mizzau, N. T. Mai, A. Sirisegaram, and M. Wilson, "Food for
   thought. What you eat depends on your sex and eating companions,"
   Appetite 53 (2009): 268-271.

8. Melinda Beck, "Eating to Live or Living to Eat," *Wall Street Journal,* July
   10, 2010, accessed February 8, 2011, http://online.wsj.com/article/SB10001
   424052748704288204575363072381955744.html.

9. "Looking for Triggers That Prompt You to Overeat," *Environmental
   Nutrition,* August 2010: Vol. 33, No. 8: 3.

Chapter 10: The Bag of Tricks

1. "Wake Up to More Muscle," *Men's Health,* April 2008: 52.

2. R. Sovik, "The Science of Breathing—The Yogic View," *Progressive Brain
   Research* 122 (2000): 491-505.

3. Heather Loeb, "Is Sleep Really Necessary?" *Men's Health,* June 2008: 137.

4. Robert E. Krout, "Music Listening to Facilitate Relaxation and Promote
   Wellness: Integrated Aspects of Our Neurophysiological Responses to
   Music," *The Arts in Psychotherapy,* 34 (2007): 134-141.

5. Marjan Farshadi and Moigan Farshadi, "Investigation of Effects of Music
   Therapy in Reducing Sleep Disorders in High School Girls," *Music Therapy
   Today VI,* no. 1 (February 2005): 110-111.

Scan this code with your smartphone to be instantly linked to *Petite Advantage Diet* bonus materials and other healthy living books and information.

You can also text keyword PETITE to READIT (732348) to be sent a link to the mobile website.